Comparative Immunobiology

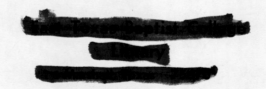

TERTIARY LEVEL BIOLOGY

A series covering selected areas of biology at advanced undergraduate level. While designed specifically for course options at this level within Universities and Polytechnics, the series will be of great value to specialists and research workers in other fields who require a knowledge of the essentials of a subject.

Other titles in the series:

Experimentation in Biology	Ridgman
Methods in Experimental Biology	Ralph
Visceral Muscle	Huddart and Hunt
Biological Membranes	Harrison and Lunt
Water and Plants	Meidner and Sheriff

Comparative Immunobiology

Margaret J. Manning, B.Sc., Ph.D.

Senior Lecturer in Zoology
University of Hull

and

Rodney J. Turner, B.Sc., Ph.D.

Research Fellow in Immunobiology
University of Hull

A HALSTED PRESS BOOK

John Wiley and Sons,

Blackie & Son Limited
Bishopbriggs
Glasgow G64 2NZ

450 Edgware Road
London W2 1EG

Published in the U.S.A. by
Halsted Press,
a Division of John Wiley and Sons Inc.,
New York

Library of Congress Cataloging in Publication Data
Manning, Margaret J
Comparative immunobiology.

Bibliography: p.
Includes index.
1. Immunology, Comparative. I. Turner, Rodney J.,
joint author. II. Title.
QR181.M34   1976   596'.02'9   75-42363
ISBN 0-470-14995-7

Printed in Great Britain by
Thomson Litho Ltd., East Kilbride, Scotland

Preface

THE APPROACH TO COMPARATIVE IMMUNOBIOLOGY WHICH WE HAVE TAKEN in this book is based on our experience in teaching the subject to undergraduates in their final year of a degree course in the Biological Sciences. The book is aimed at this level and is written primarily for students who wish to know something about the immune system, particularly its evolutionary and comparative aspects, while not necessarily intending to specialize in Immunobiology. Hopefully, it may also provide an introduction to the phylogeny of the immune response for those who already have some advanced knowledge of other branches of Immunobiology.

We are indebted to Dr. William M. Baldwin III of the Department of Microbiology, University of Rochester, U.S.A., who drew the Figures, and whose combination of artistic skills and immunological insight makes a most valuable contribution to the book. Other colleagues in the University of Rochester, particularly Dr. Nicholas Cohen, have given helpful advice and criticism. Our sincere thanks go to our co-workers in the University of Hull, Dr. John D. Horton and Mrs. Trudy L. Horton, now in the University of Durham, for their excellent photographs and for allowing us to use a previously unpublished electron micrograph (figure 1.7b); and to Mrs. Andrea Randall and Miss Madeleine Collie, who provided the photographs used in figures 6.2 and 6.8, and who assisted us in many other ways. We are also grateful to our publishers for their help and encouragement.

Lastly, but most importantly, we owe a great debt to the many immunologists from whose studies we have drawn our information. They have not been cited, since detailed references would be inappropriate in a book of this sort, but many of the original papers can be traced through the books and review articles listed in the Further Reading section.

Contents

CHAPTER ONE

THE IMMUNE SYSTEM

1.1. Introduction

This first chapter provides a brief survey of the immune system. It is intended as a background to subsequent chapters in which we shall discuss the immunobiology of the separate vertebrate classes—largely from a phylogenetic aspect, but also in terms of its relevance to the animals' overall structure, physiology and way of life. For more detailed information on basic immunology the reader is referred to several excellent textbooks listed in the Further Reading section on page 174.

Not surprisingly, current concepts of the immune system are based largely on studies of man and other mammals (and to some extent on birds, notably the chicken), and much of the evidence which we shall discuss in Chapter 1 centres on these animals. Immunological mechanisms may, however, be less complex and therefore more easily understood at lower levels of phylogeny, and some groups offer specific experimental advantages: the temperature-dependence of poikilothermic animals may, for instance, be manipulated to slow down or speed up critical events, and the free-living early stages of amphibians are more readily accessible for experimentation than amniote embryos. Besides these practical advantages, a phylogenetic perspective may enable us to distinguish those features of the immune system which are of central importance from detailed variants which are the end-products of adaptive radiation and which, while interesting in themselves, may be relevant only to particular classes or may even differ from one species to another.

1.2. The basis of immunity

The defence mechanisms of the body serve to inactivate or eliminate foreign invaders, particularly pathogenic micro-organisms and their

1

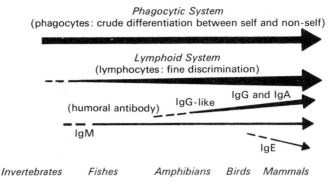

Figure 1.1. Phylogeny of internal defence mechanisms
IgM, IgG, etc., indicate different antibody classes (see section 1.4.2).

products, by methods such as phagocytosis (engulfment), encapsulation, and the production of various soluble substances. To these phylogenetically ancient defences, the vertebrates add a highly specific immune system which is based at the molecular level on antibody molecules (immunoglobulins) and at the cellular level on lymphocytes (figure 1.1). The origins of the vertebrate system from its invertebrate ancestry are discussed in Chapter 2.

The immune system involves a sophisticated recognition of non-self and is characterized by memory, specificity and diversity. Substances which elicit an immune response are called *immunogens* or *antigens*. The responses may be (i) *humoral*, with the production of circulating antibodies which possess specificity towards the antigen which elicited their production, and/or (ii) *cell-mediated*, in which the effectors are the cells themselves. Both types of response evoke a proliferation of lymphocytes which recognize the antigen and react specifically to it and, in both types of response, the reaction to a repeated exposure (the secondary response) is different from that occurring after the first encounter with the same antigen. The secondary response is usually more vigorous than the primary response. This is the basis for the actively acquired immunity which occurs naturally after exposure to infection, or which may be deliberately induced by immunization procedures in which the pathogen is presented in some relatively harmless form, such as in poliomyelitis vaccination, where either killed viruses or attenuated organisms are used. Secondary responses are specific: the body can discriminate between one antigen and another, and gives a secondary response only to an antigen which is the same as the one previously encountered.

1.3. Immunoglobulins and antigen recognition

1.3.1. *The immunoglobulin molecule*

Immunoglobulins are key molecules in vertebrate immunology. They are present in the body fluids, e.g. as antibodies circulating in the gamma globulin fraction of the serum. They also occur on the surface of lymphocytes, and it is now thought that these membrane-associated immunoglobulins are the agents by which the cell recognizes the antigen.

The immunoglobulin molecule itself is based on one or more units comprising four polypeptide chains, of which two are identical heavy chains and two are identical light chains (the 2H-2L molecule, figure 1.2). In all the immunoglobulins analysed so far, the molecules have been shown to possess variations in their amino acid sequences in approximately the first 110 residues of the light and heavy polypeptide chains of the N-terminal section (the variable region). These variations can account for the large number of antibodies which an animal is capable of producing. Thus there may well be some 10^4 or 10^5 immunoglobulins, each with a different amino acid sequence in the variable region. The three-dimensional structure of this part of the immunoglobulin molecule allows for binding of a complementary site, known as an *epitope* or *determinant*, situated on the antigen.

One immunoglobulin molecule is specific only for one type of antigenic determinant. However, there may be many different determinants on a single antigen, so that the antigen can elicit synthesis of many different antibody populations (figure 1.3). Antigens are large molecules (proteins, glycoproteins, lipoproteins, polysaccharides, lipopolysaccharides or nucleic acids); among the more important antigens are those which are part of the surface membrances of cells or micro-organisms.

1.3.2. *Histocompatibility antigens*

The body's own cells have important antigenic characteristics. The first well-documented example of recognizable specific differences in external cell surfaces was provided by human erythrocytes, where inherited antigenic patterns determine the blood groups. Other antigenic sites occur in association with the nucleated blood cells and the cells of other tissues (liver, kidney, skin, etc.). These histocompatibility antigens are glycoproteins of the cell surface; they are of prime importance in transplantation and, like the blood groups, are genetically controlled. Genetically identical

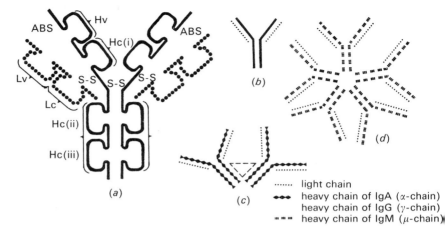

light chain
heavy chain of IgA (α-chain)
heavy chain of IgG (γ-chain)
heavy chain of IgM (μ-chain)

Figure 1.2.   Structural arrangements of the polypeptide chains of anti-body molecules (immunoglobulins)

(a) *Schematic diagram of the structure of an immunoglobulin molecule of the IgG class.*

The molecule consists of four polypeptide chains, two identical heavy (H) chains (solid lines) of molecular weight about 50,000, and two identical light (L) chains (dotted lines) of molecular weight about 25,000. These are joined by interchain disulphide bonds (S–S). The variable N-terminal regions of a light chain and a heavy chain (Lv and Hv respectively) form a site which can combine with an antigenic determinant (the antigen binding site, ABS). The 2H-2L IgG molecule has two such sites. Intrachain disulphide bonds form loops in the polypeptide chains, each representing a single domain of some 110 amino acids. A linear periodicity in amino acid sequences suggests repeating domains in the constant part of the immunoglobulin molecule (Lc in the light chain and Hc(i), Hc(ii), Hc(iii) in the heavy chain), probably with some specialization in biological functions.

Partly from Roitt, I. (1974), *Essential Immunology*, 2nd ed., Blackwell Scientific Publications, Oxford (with modifications).

(b), (c), (d). *Comparative structures of immunoglobulins of different classes (see section 1.4.2).*

(b) The IgG molecule (simplified from diagram a). IgG comprises a single 2H-2L unit.

(c) The IgA molecule. IgA frequently occurs as a dimer (two 2H-2L units). It is shown here in the form found in secretory fluids, i.e. with an added secretory piece (shown diagrammatically as a triangle).

(d) The IgM molecule. IgM is a large polymeric immunoglobulin with multiple binding sites, usually a pentamer (five 2H-2L units).

Note that the differences between immunoglobulins of the different classes are governed by their different heavy chains (the γ-chains, α-chains and μ-chains of IgG, IgA and IgM respectively).

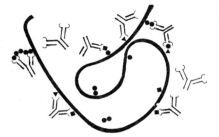

antigenic determinants

- ■ determinant (a)
- ● determinant (b)
- ▶ determinant (c)
- ◆ determinant (a) showing cross-reactivity with an immunoglobulin directed against (c) (bottom left of diagram)

Figure 1.3. Diagrammatic representation of an antigen molecule
Many different antigenic determinants may be present on a single large antigen molecule. These determinants are small three-dimensional configurations (for example, some 8–12 amino acids of a polypeptide chain); in figure 1.3 they are shown as symbols placed on a thick continuous line which represents the antigen molecule. An antibody-synthesizing cell produces antibody to only one antigenic determinant. An antigen such as that shown in the diagram elicits production of a variety of immunoglobulins from different cells which recognize different determinants on its molecule. These immunoglobulins differ in their antigen binding sites—as is indicated diagrammatically on the 2H-2L antibody structures shown in figure 1.3. Flexibility of the immunoglobulin chains permits bivalent combination, as is figured for antigenic determinant (b) in the top left and top right parts of the diagram. Effective antigenic determinants are those which are exposed on the surface of the antigen molecule.

individuals will accept grafts from each other (*syngeneic grafts*); however, members of the same species but of different genetic constitution will not. Their grafts (*allogeneic grafts*, also called *allografts* or *homografts*) are normally rejected with greater or lesser speed and intensity, according to (i) the amount of genetic disparity and (ii) whether they differ with respect to loci controlling "strong" histocompatibility antigens, i.e. those which provoke a strong allograft reaction. Grafts from animals of a different species are termed *xenografts*, and grafts made when self-tissues are grafted back on to the original donor are called *autografts*; the former are rejected, the latter are retained.

It is now known that genes which code for the rapid rejection of allogeneic grafts and for "strong" histocompatibility antigens, such as those of the important transplantation systems H-2 in mice and HL-A in man, are closely linked into a major histocompatibility system. This complex is genetically determined by a series of closely linked genes which control not only the major histocompatibility systems but also other immune reactions, including genetic regulation of immune responsiveness to certain well-defined antigens (the immune response (Ir) gene).

1.3.3. *Clonal selection and memory*

It is believed that the lymphocyte plays a fundamental role as the carrier of surface-associated immunoglobulins which act as receptor sites for antigen recognition. Furthermore, according to the widely accepted theory of clonal selection, each lymphocyte has the genetic information to make immunoglobulin molecules of one specificity only, and there is a diverse population of lymphocytes, each with the ability to produce its own particular amino acid sequence in the variable region of the molecule. It is not yet known whether the genetic basis of this diversity depends on the possession of a very large number of genes to code for the variable portions, or whether a small number of germ-line genes undergo randomized somatic mutation during the development of an individual. The diversity means that a large number of antigens can be recognized. However, any one receptor site may be relatively infrequent in the lymphocytic population; it is therefore of adaptive significance that encounter with antigen triggers proliferation of the specifically reactive cells and so increases their number (figure 1.4).

Engagement of antigen with the specific immunoglobulin receptor site on the surface of a lymphocyte initiates a series of events which leads via mitotic divisions to effector cell differentiation. In humoral immune responses, these effectors are antibody-producing cells (called *plasma cells*); they possess highly differentiated cytoplasmic machinery for the manufacture and secretion of the specific antibody expressed by their clone. Not all the progeny of the clone become effectors, however. Some revert to their lymphocytic role as carriers of the specific antigen receptors; these are *memory cells*. Their numerical build-up alone could account for secondary responses, but it is probable that they have also altered qualitatively and, as sensitized cells, differ from virgin lymphocytes which have not yet encountered antigen.

The formation of clones of memory cells will result in a relative increase of receptor sites for antigens previously encountered, many of which are likely to be those that occur frequently in the environment. The animal therefore acquires, by cumulative immunological experience, a well-adjusted force to which recruits (in the form of lymphocytes with randomly generated new receptors) continue to be added. The newly-entering lymphocytes are then available to replace clones, whose lifespans are finite, and to deal with fresh antigens which the animal may meet for the first time. New formation of lymphocytes falls off markedly in the mature animal as the organs concerned, notably the thymus, become involuted. This limitation may prevent undue crowding-out of patterns which have already been selected during the life of the animal, and which may help to adapt it to its environment.

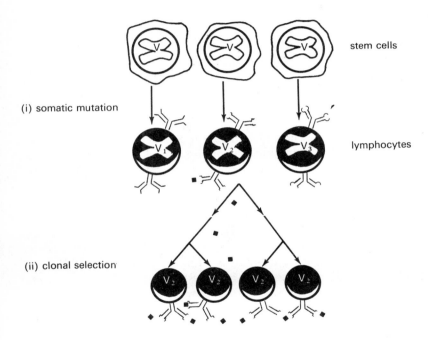

Figure 1.4.   Antibody diversity and clonal selection

(i) One theory of antibody diversity, that of somatic mutation, postulates that a basic gene or a small number of germ line genes (V) undergo randomized somatic mutation to give different genes (V_1, V_2, V_3, etc.) yielding a diverse population of lymphocytes, each with the genes coding for one specific antibody. This antibody forms the receptor (indicated in the diagram as 2H-2L immunoglobulin on the lymphocyte surface) by which the cell recognizes an antigenic determinant.

(ii) Encounter with the specific antigenic determinant (represented as a black square) triggers the cell to proliferate (clonal selection) and possibly to differentiate into an effector cell secreting the specific antibody.

1.4. Protective role of antibody

1.4.1. *Defence against foreign organisms*

There are a number of ways in which antibodies help to render harmless any pathogens which invade the body:

(i) Toxins, such as the soluble exotoxins of bacteria, may be neutralized by direct combination with antibody.

(ii) Neutralization of viruses by antibody inhibits the ability of the virus to infect the body's cells.

(iii) Some organisms such as metazoan parasites and spores may elicit formation of a special class of antibody called IgE. IgE binds to mast cells (basophilic granulocytes present in the tissues) and, on subsequent contact with specific antigen, releases from these cells potent agents such as histamine (figure 1.5*a*). These pharmacological products cause smooth-muscle contraction, capillary dilation and tear formation, and possibly aid expulsion by physical displacement of the parasite.

(iv) Micro-organisms may be clumped together to form non-invasive aggregates. This agglutination can occur because immunoglobulin molecules have two or more combining sites which can link adjacent antigenic particles (figure 1.5*b*).

(v) Antigen-antibody complexes can activate serum proteins known as *complement*. If the antigen is a cell of some kind (e.g. a bacterium), this generates membrane damage which results in rupture (lysis) and kills the cell (figure 1.5*c*).

(vi) Coating with specific antibody is often necessary before organisms can adhere to macrophages and be ingested by them. This process (opsonization) is enhanced by part of the complement system (figure 1.6).

(vii) Activation of complement by antigen-antibody complexes releases complement fractions which are chemotactic for polymorph neutrophils (small phagocytes) and which elicit inflammatory reactions.

(viii) The final pathway for elimination of the neutralized toxins, killed micro-organisms and the various complexes which result from immuno-logical activity, is through phagocytosis.

It is apparent that antibodies themselves are not the agents of significant biological damage, but that they act against invaders in conjunction with non-specific effector mechanisms—in particular through the complement system and through phagocytosis. Complement comprises at least 9 normal serum factors which act sequentially. In the usual (classical) responses, the sequence is initiated by antigen-antibody complexes. However there are alternative, but less efficient, pathways which do not involve antibody

a
mast cell degranulation

b
agglutination

c
complement-mediated cell lysis

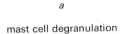
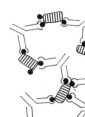
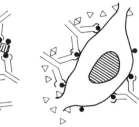
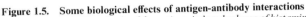

Figure 1.5.   Some biological effects of antigen-antibody interactions
(a) *Mediation by IgE antibody of the antigen-induced release of histamine from mast cells.*

Immunoglobulins of the class IgE have the property of binding to tissue cells. When IgE antibodies attached to a mast cell (as shown in figure 1.5a) interact with specific antigen (represented by black squares), they mediate the release of histamine and other agents (indicated by dots) from the mast cell granules.

(b) *Antigen agglutination by antibody.*

Agglutination is brought about by the linking of particulate antigens such as erythrocytes or bacteria (striped in diagram) by the antigen binding regions of an immunoglobulin molecule which combine with antigenic determinants (shown as solid circles) on adjacent particles. The immunoglobulin molecules are represented in the diagram as IgG molecules (2H-2L). IgM with its multiple binding sites (see figure 1.2d) is even more effective in bringing about agglutination.

(c) *Cell lysis mediated by antibody and complement.*

Figure 1.5c shows a cell (the antigen) with its nucleus (striped) and surface antigenic determinants (solid circles). Combination of specific antibody with antigenic determinants can result in fixation of the first component of the complement series. Complement activation involves the Hc(ii) domain of the heavy chain (see figure 1.2) of the immunoglobulin molecule (depicted in the diagram by the attachment of complement (double triangle) to this part of the 2H-2L molecule). Complement activation sets in train a sequence of events in the complement series, producing an amplification (cascade) effect—indicated by triangles—and terminating in the appearance of functional holes in the cell membrane (shown at the top and bottom of the diagram), with subsequent lysis and cell death. Complement is fixed by IgG and IgM antibodies. IgM is highly efficient and can activate the full complement series by a single hit; IgG fixes complement only when two or more immunoglobulin molecules are bound to closely adjacent sites on the antigen (as is indicated in diagram 1.5c on the left).

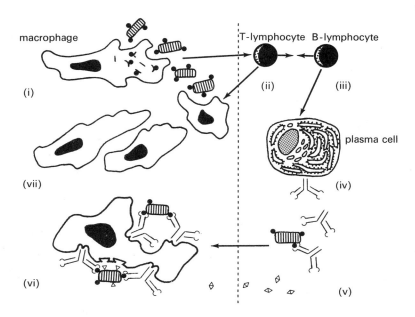

Figure 1.6 indicates some of the interrelationships between macrophage activities and the immune functions of lymphocytes.

(i)   Macrophages are involved in trapping and processing antigens. [The antigen is depicted as a cell (striped) with antigenic determinants (solid circles).]

(ii)   Antigen processed by macrophages can stimulate T-lymphocytes (see section 1.8).

(iii)   T-lymphocytes co-operate with B-lymphocytes in antibody production to certain antigens (see section 1.8.4).

(iv)   Stimulated B-lymphocytes may undergo division and differentiation to produce antibody-forming cells (plasma cells). These cells have the cytoplasmic machinery for synthesizing and secreting antibody. (The endoplasmic reticulum, with attached ribosomal (RNA) granules, and the Golgi apparatus are depicted in diagram (iv).)

(v)   Secreted antibody coats the antigen. In addition, the complement system (double triangles) may be activated.

(vi)   The antibody-coated antigen shows an enhanced ability to adhere to macrophages; this facilitates its engulfment and destruction. This increased phagocytosis (opsonization) is brought about partly through IgG molecules which in combination with antigen develop a heightened binding affinity for specific sites on the surface of macrophages (indicated at the top of diagram (vi)). In addition, macrophages have binding sites for complement when but by which at least some of the complement mechanism can be activated; these may be of older (possibly pre-vertebrate) phylogenetic origin. Parts of more ancient defence mechanisms are thus by no means obsolete; nevertheless, the severity of certain immunodeficiency diseases indicates the importance of the immune system—at least to the higher vertebrates.

The antigen-antibody reactions which have their protective role *in vivo* can be studied in the laboratory by tests which include:

(i) The precipitation of soluble antigens by antibodies (termed *precipitins*).

(ii) The agglutination of cells or of antigen-coated particles by specific agglutinating antibodies (erythrocytes are frequently used in these tests).

(iii) Complement fixation and lysis (again, erythrocytes are frequently used as indicators).

(iv) Methods using labelled antibodies, e.g. those labelled with a fluorescent dye.

(v) Antigen-binding techniques, e.g. using radioactive antigen.

(vi) Tests based on the neutralization of biological activities.

1.4.2. *Role of antibody classes*

The variable portion of the immunoglobulin molecule determines its specificity. Other important biological properties are governed by the structure of the heavy chain (figure 1.2), and this determines a diversity of roles for immunoglobulins which have similar specificities. In man the major immunoglobulin (Ig) classes, grouped in accordance with their heavy-chain characteristics, are IgG, IgA, IgM, IgD and IgE. In each immunoglobulin class, molecules can be recognized with two different antigenic forms of light chain (kappa and lambda) which have been shown to possess distinct primary structures. Also, the whole range of combining specificities are probably represented throughout the classes.

---

this is present in the form of the modified third component (C_3)— indicated by triangles; this allows for the immune adherence of antigen-antibody-complement complexes, as shown at the bottom of diagram (vi).

(vii) When sensitized T-lymphocytes are stimulated, they may release non-immunoglobulin agents, some of which can affect the activity of macrophages (see section 1.8.4). Migration of macrophages may be inhibited with the result that these cells can accumulate at the site of the reaction. In addition, T-lymphocyte factors may render the macrophage more effective in killing ingested organisms.

Among the activities which probably depend upon the class of antibody are:

(i) The ability of the antigen-antibody complex to fix complement (present in IgM and most IgG antibodies).

(ii) Attachment to mast cells (IgE).

(iii) The distribution in the body. IgG is the most abundant immuno-globulin, particularly in the extra-vascular body fluids; antibodies of this class can cross the placenta. IgM remains largely within the blood circulation except where vascular permeability is increased locally, as in inflammation. IgA is released into the sero-mucous secretions and occurs in saliva, tears, mammary-gland secretions and gut secretions.

(iv) The state of polymerization. IgM exists as a five-fold polymer of the basic 2H-2L unit, while the IgA in the external secretions occurs as a dimer. The polymeric IgM molecules with their multiple antigen-binding sites are efficient agglutinating and complement-fixing agents; they tend to appear early in the response to infections.

Immunoglobulin polymers incorporate additional polypeptide chains known as J (joining) chains. High and low-molecular-weight immuno-globulins are sometimes referred to by their sedimentation coefficients; e.g. IgM is 19S immunoglobulin, IgG is 7S immunoglobulin. Experi-mentally they are often distinguished by their sensitivity to 2-mercapto-ethanol, since quite often the 19S antibody is sensitive to inactivation by this chemical, while the 7S antibody is resistant. This is not invariable however; in some species, the 7S as well as the 19S antibody is sensitive to 2-mercaptoethanol, conversely part of the 19S fraction is sometimes resistant. In the response to many antigens, 7S antibody substitutes for 19S during the time course of the reaction.

1.5. Cell-mediated immunity

Antigens which readily reach the lymphoid organs are likely to cause humoral antibody production, whereas those which gain access less readily may instead be reached and recognized by lymphoid cells which them-selves circulate; such antigens tend to elicit cell-mediated immunity. In fact, many natural antigens produce both types of response, but cell-mediated immunity predominates in the following circumstances:

(i) In response to histocompatibility antigens. The transplantation of foreign tissues provides a good example, although an unnatural one, of an antigen which elicits a cellular response (figure 1.7a and b). An allograft of skin, for example, will induce a reaction which is manifested, in the

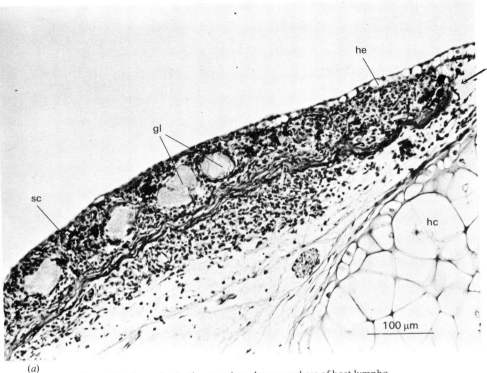

(a)

Figure 1.7. In graft rejection reactions, large numbers of host lymphocytes infiltrate the graft. This cellular immune response is clearly
demonstrated in transplantation experiments such as those in the
amphibian *Xenopus laevis* illustrated.

Figure 1.7a shows a histological section through an allograft of
toadlet skin on the tenth day after transplantation on to an immunologically competent host (a *X. laevis* larva with a well-differentiated
lymphoid system). The graft is undergoing rejection in a cellular
immune reaction involving many host lymphocytes. These lymphocytes, with their small deeply-stained nuclei, are conspicuous both
within the transplanted tissue and beneath it. The glands of the graft
(gl) are being destroyed. The stratum compactum of the graft cutis
(sc) assumes a wavy appearance as lymphocytes penetrate between its
fibres. New host epidermis (he) is growing over the edge of the graft
region; this is seen in the upper right of the field (the upper edge of the
graft is marked with an arrow). The tissue in the lower right of the
photograph is host cartilage (hc).

From Horton, J. D. (1969), "Ontogeny of the Immune Response to
Skin Allografts in relation to Lymphoid Organ Development in the
Amphibian *Xenopus laevis* Daudin", *Journal of Experimental Zoology*,
170, 449–466.

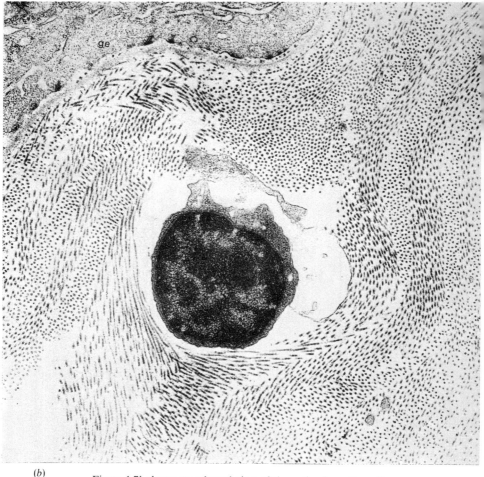

(b)

Figure 1.7b shows an enlarged view of the cutis of an allograft on *Xenopus laevis*. This electron micrograph shows a single lymphocyte penetrating between the graft fibres, most of which are cut obliquely or transversely. Part of an epithelial cell of the graft (ge) is seen in the upper left of the field. The picture illustrates some of the features of the small lymphocyte, a cell which typically shows a rounded nucleus with dense marginated chromatin masses and a high nucleo-cytoplasmic ratio. The sparse cytoplasm is seen here as a thin rim around the nucleus on the upper and right-hand sides of the cell. Magnification × 15,000.

Courtesy of Dr. J. D. Horton. We would like to thank Mrs. Janice Mundy of the University of Hull for help with the electron microscopy.

first instance, by the occurrence of lymphoid cells within and around the graft. It has been suggested that the role of these circulating lymphocytes is that of surveillance, and that cell-mediated immunity arose in phylogeny as a means of patrolling the tissues for any of the body's cells which may be changed in their antigenic characteristics. Antigenic changes may be detected on the surface of tumour cells, and this may be the means of recognizing and destroying potentially neoplastic tissue.

(ii) In reactions known as *delayed hypersensitivities*. Thus some plant substances and various drugs cause local cellular immune reactions, e.g. the contact sensitivity which is produced when certain chemicals are applied to the skin.

(iii) In response to various fungi and to some protozoan and metazoan parasites, especially those which establish themselves within the tissues.

(iv) In situations where the pathogen is inaccessible for destruction by circulating antibody, because it rapidly becomes intracellular within the host. This group includes bacilli, such as those of tuberculosis and leprosy which continue to grow within the cytoplasm of macrophages following their uptake by these cells.

(v) In response to some viruses, especially such as those of smallpox which rapidly become intracellular. It is possible that entry of the virus results in new antigens appearing on the cell surface, with subsequent destruction of the infected cell by a mechanism similar to that of graft rejection.

1.6. Antigen-specific non-reactivity

1.6.1. *Immunological tolerance*

Immunological memory need not necessarily be positive, in the sense that it leads to increased reactivity. On the contrary, it may under some circumstances be expressed as a specific failure to respond, i.e. immunological tolerance. This is readily demonstrated in chimaeras, animals which carry live cells from another individual and which are specifically tolerant to such cells. The situation was analysed experimentally by Medawar and his colleagues, who showed that mice inoculated with allogeneic cells early in development tolerated a skin graft from the same donor applied later in life. Grafts from unrelated donors were rejected in normal fashion, thus demonstrating the specificity of acquired immunological tolerance.

Immunologically tolerant chimaeras have been produced during the early stages of development by several methods:

(i) By shared blood circulation. This occurs naturally through placental anastomoses, notably in some cattle twins (where this type of tolerance was first demonstrated by Owen). It can also be achieved by joining two animals experimentally by parabiosis, as in chick embryos or larval amphibians (see section 5.1.2).

(ii) By injection of cell suspensions (as described above) or by means of large grafts made between embryos (figure 1.8); in some amphibians it is possible to exchange half embryos.

(iii) By experimentally assembling the blastomeres from two embryos as in allophenic mice.

These experiments have in common the fact that massive exposure to the foreign antigen occurred before the maturation of a competent immune system. It has been suggested that such early encounters with antigen have the effect, not of inducing clonal proliferation, but on the contrary, of killing or in some way suppressing any lymphocytes which are capable of recognizing the antigens concerned, and that this is the means of self-recognition which ensures that the body's own tissues do not normally become the subject of immunological attack.

While tolerance to histocompatibility antigens has a special significance early in ontogenetic development, the phenomenon of tolerance extends to the adult state and to non-living materials. Adult mice, for example, can be made tolerant to foreign serum proteins. Factors which influence the decision whether a lymphocyte which encounters antigen will follow the pathway to immunity or to tolerance include the dose, the degree of foreignness, the physical state of the antigen and the method of presentation, as well as the maturity of the recipient. It has been suggested that antigens are tolerogenic if they react directly with lymphocytes, and that to elicit a positive immune response they must first be processed by macrophages (large phagocytes). Uptake by macrophages occurs more readily if the antigen is in an aggregated or particulate form.

1.6.2. Enhancement

In the classical model of transplantation tolerance, specific lymphocytes are thought to be irreversibly inactivated. However, it has long been recognized that the prolonged survival of tumours and other tissues may, under appropriate circumstances, be brought about by the active production of humoral factors (enhancing antibodies). These may mask

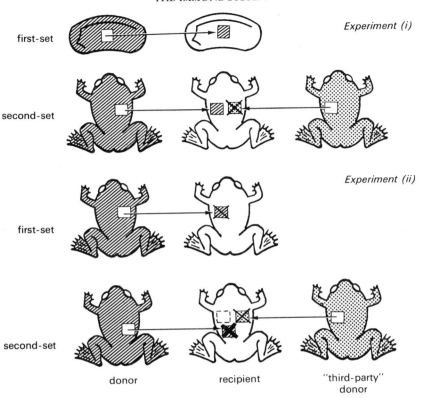

Figure 1.8. Tolerance induction and immunity in frogs

The outcome of a second-set (i.e. second time) exposure to an allograft may be either specific tolerance or specific immunity, according to the state of maturity of the animal at the time when first exposure to the antigen occurred.

In experiment (i), a large graft of flank tissue is transferred from an embryo at the neurula stage of development to another embryo of the same age. The animals are allowed to grow into frogs, then a second graft (a skin graft) from the same donor is applied. This graft is tolerated, i.e. it is retained indefinitely and is not rejected. The tolerance is specific, as demonstrated by the ability of the recipient to reject grafts taken from "third-party" donors, i.e. animals unrelated to the original donor.

In experiment (ii), first-set grafting is postponed until the animal is mature. In this case a second-set graft from the same donor is rejected; furthermore, it is rejected more rapidly than the first-set graft, i.e. it elicits positive second-set immunity. Again, the response is specific, as demonstrated by the slower rejection (within first-set times) of grafts taken from a third-party donor.

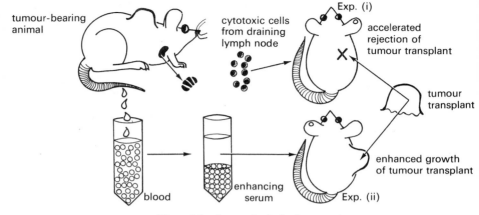

Figure 1.9.   Immunological enhancement
Figure 1.9 illustrates the role of enhancing antibodies in promoting
the survival of transplanted tumours. Cytotoxic cells capable of
destroying tumour cells may be present in the tumour-bearing animal
(as demonstrated in exp. (i)). They may, however, be prevented from
exerting their function by the presence of serum factors (shown in
exp. (ii)). These factors are specific antibodies, or possibly immune
complexes of transplantation antigens and antibody. They may prevent
delivery of antigens in immunogenic form to the lymphoid cells, and/or
they may block the antigenic sites of the graft, thus preventing its
destruction by sensitized cytotoxic cells (as depicted in figure 1.9).

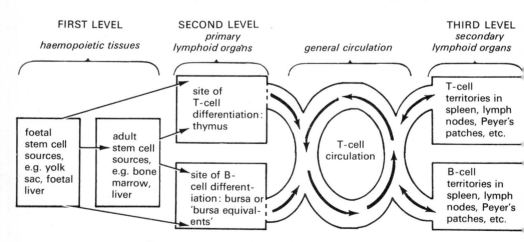

Figure 1.10.   Differentiation pathways of immunocompetent cells
Diagram to show roles of the lymphoid organs in the differentiation
of T-cell and B-cell lymphocytes.

the antigens of transplanted tissues, thereby either stopping them from immunizing the recipient or preventing their destruction by effector lymphocytes. This form of graft survival can be passively transferred to another animal by means of serum (figure 1.9). The possibility should be borne in mind that this mechanism (and/or a central failure) may operate in some cases of chimaerism and of transplantation tolerance, and that some instances of prolonged graft survival may involve a delicate balance between enhancement and positive cytotoxic immune reactions.

1.7. Sequence of differentiation

1.7.1. *Role of lymphoid organs*

Haemopoietic tissues

Stem-cells of the immune system are housed in haemopoietic (blood-forming) tissues such as those of the embryonic yolk sac, the foetal liver, spleen and bone marrow. In the adult mammal, the bone marrow is the main source of stem-cells. The stem-cell pool represents the first level of differentiation (figure 1.10) and is believed to comprise a self-perpetuating population of multipotent cells. These are common haemopoietic stem-cells for erythrocytes, granulocytes, etc., as well as for lymphocytes. Haemopoietic tissue is closely associated with the vascular system, and occurs in sinusoidal areas where cells can move readily into and out of the blood.

Primary lymphoid organs

The secondary level of differentiation occurs in the primary lymphoid organs, e.g. the thymus and bursa of Fabricius. Within the primary lymphoid organs, stem-cells divide and develop into immunologically competent lymphocytes. The brisk mitotic activity which accompanies this phase of differentiation strongly suggests that this is the time when diversity within the lymphocytic population is generated. However, it is still not known for certain exactly when the lymphocyte acquires its antigen-specific receptors. After several cycles of division, some lymphocytes leave the primary lymphoid organs, and these either circulate around the body or settle in secondary lymphoid tissue.

The primary lymphoid organs originate as epithelial anlagen, the

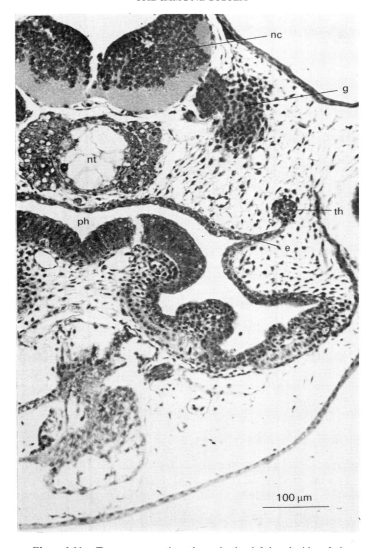

Figure 1.11. Transverse section through the left-hand side of the pharyngeal region of a 3-day-old amphibian larva (*Xenopus laevis*) in the region of the second pharyngeal pouch. The section shows the developing thymus which at this early stage is an epithelial bud still attached to the pharyngeal epithelium from which it originates. e, pharyngeal epithelium; g, nerve ganglion; nc, nerve cord; nt, notochord; ph, pharynx; th, thymus.

thymus as a bud from the pharyngeal epithelium (figure 1.11) and the bursa of Fabricius as a dorsal diverticulum of the cloaca in birds (figure 8.4). The epithelium forms a framework of branched cells infiltrated by lymphocytes. The possession of this epithelial component is a feature which distinguishes the primary lymphoid organs from the other tissues of the immune system.

Because the thymus develops from the pharyngeal epithelium, and because important endocrine organs such as the thyroid and parathyroid also develop from this same general area, it has long been suspected that the thymus might secrete humoral substances. There is indeed a likelihood that the thymic epithelial cells release factors which affect the differentiation of lymphoid cells, perhaps mainly those in their immediate environment, but possibly extra-thymic cells as well. The insertion into the immune system of internally-regulated primary lymphoid organs is of significance, since these provide a necessary safeguard against possible exhaustive overstimulation by external factors in a pathway where, throughout life, the final stage of differentiation is governed by exogenous antigen.

Secondary lymphoid organs

The third level of functional differentiation occurs in the secondary lymphoid organs. In these organs, in contrast to the primary lymphoid tissues, lymphocytic proliferation is almost entirely antigen-driven. Thus encounter of a lymphocyte with an antigen to which it can respond usually leads to a further phase of differentiation. This begins with enlargement of the lymphocyte to form a blast cell. The cytoplasm acquires a high ribosome content, and therefore stains deep pink with the dye pyronin, i.e. the cell becomes pyroninophilic. There follows a series of mitotic divisions which produce (i) effector cells of the immune system and (ii) sensitized lymphocytes which form memory cells.

The secondary lymphoid organs have a complex structure, with arrangements for trapping antigen and ensuring that it is presented in suitable form to cells capable of reacting to it. They include areas for circulation of cells of the immune system within an anatomical framework which increases the opportunities for the chance meeting of antigen and antigen-reactive cell. They accommodate the proliferating lymphoid populations which result from antigenic stimulation, house the developing effector cells, and provide for the release of their products. In the mammal, the organs concerned are the lymph nodes, which receive antigen mainly from the lymph; the spleen which is situated in the blood circulation; tonsils, Peyer's patches, appendix and solitary nodules of the gut wall; lymphatic nodules in the respiratory, urinary and genital tracts, and scattered lymphoid tissue elsewhere in the body.

1.8. B-cells and T-cells

1.8.1. *Ontogeny of B-cells and T-cells*

It is now known that the functional dichotomy between humoral immunity and cell-mediated responses extends to the cellular level, and that different cell lineages are involved (the B-cells and T-cells). Furthermore these separate lineages can be traced back to their origins in different primary lymphoid organs. Thus establishment of a normal population of immunologically competent T-cells depends on the presence of an intact thymus. The B-cell lineage, on the other hand, is independent of the thymus; in birds, an intact bursa of Fabricius is required for the establishment of B-cell functions.

1.8.2. *Differences between B-cells and T-cells*

Although lymphocytes of the B-cell and T-cell populations are not readily separated by histological criteria, it is possible to distinguish between them on other grounds. On B-lymphocytes, surface immunoglobulins are readily demonstrated using an antiserum to the immunoglobulin; on T-lymphocytes they are more difficult to detect. For the T-lymphocytes of the mouse there is a useful marker: this is the surface antigen theta (thy-1) which can be identified by means of anti-theta antiserum raised in mice of a different strain. Most of the long-lived lymphocytes which circulate in the blood and lymph are T-cells bearing this theta antigen. T-cells are less "sticky" than B-cells (they adhere less readily to surfaces) and they are more negatively charged. Certain mitogens can stimulate lymphocytes in a non-specific way; of these, phytohaemagglutinin (PHA) stimulates only T-cells, while bacterial lipopolysaccharide (LPS) stimulates only B-cells.

1.8.3. *Territories of B-cells and T-cells*

The dichotomy between humoral immunity and cell-mediated responses is also reflected in the anatomy of the secondary lymphoid organs.

Antigens which elicit antibody production stimulate certain areas, such as the cortex of the lymph node (figure 1.12). These are places where antigen is trapped and B-cells settle. In these regions there are compact lymphoid follicles where antigen is held on specialized dendritic processes of reticular cells. This form of antigen-trapping probably depends on the presence of antibody. Functionally it brings the antigen into intimate contact with the

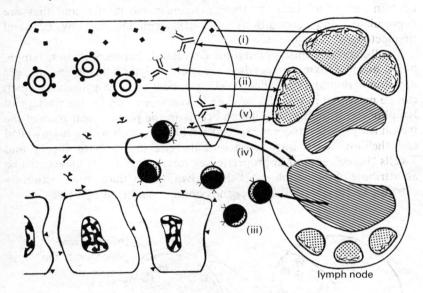

lymph node

Figure 1.12. Lymph node responses in humoral and cell-mediated immunity

Soluble antigens (represented as black squares) (i) and particulate antigens such as micro-organisms (circles with the antigenic deter-minants shown as solid circles) (ii) enter the blood or lymph and are carried to secondary lymphoid organs (e.g. via lymphatic vessels to the regional lymph nodes as depicted on the right) where they reach antigen-trapping areas in the B-cell territories (e.g. in the cortex of the lymph node (dotted)). The B-cell areas then enlarge (as indicated at the top of the lymph node), and circulating antibodies are produced.

Antigens, such as those which cause delayed hypersensitivity responses, and those of tumours and skin grafts (shown at the bottom left with antigenic determinants represented as triangles) reach the lymphoid organs less readily and instead may be recognized by T-lymphocytes which themselves circulate (iii). Antigen and stimulated T-lymphocytes (iv) then cause enlargement of the paracortical areas of the lymph node (i.e. the T-cell territory, indicated by stripes), with the production of effector T-cells. (In addition, some graft antigen may reach the B-cell areas and elicit antibody production (v)).

B-lymphocytes, and causes their enlargement and division; the areas of proliferation are called *germinal centres*. On the other hand, with antigens which produce cell-mediated responses, the enlargement and proliferation (in this case of T-lymphocytes) occurs in a different part of the organ, e.g. the paracortical zone of lymph nodes and the periarteriolar sheaths of the spleen (figure 1.13). These thymus-dependent areas have been shown to contain cells which bear the theta antigen in the mouse, and they are depopulated under conditions of T-cell depletion, e.g. by neonatal thymectomy.

T-cells are a mobile population circulating between tissues, lymph, blood and the thymus-dependent areas of the lymphoid organs in their function of immune surveillance. Many appear to have a life-span which can be measured in months, or even in years. A route for the passage of lymphocytes from blood to lymph occurs in the paracortical zone of the lymph nodes, where there are specialized blood vessels with a high-walled endothelium. When introduced into the circulation, both B-cells and T-cells "home" to their appropriate territories. This ability appears to be an attribute of the lymphocytes themselves, rather than an attraction by extrinsic factors; it probably depends on their surface properties.

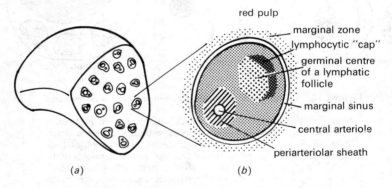

Figure 1.13. Schematic diagram of the rat spleen

(a) Spleen cut in half to show the white pulp areas lying within the red pulp.

(b) Enlarged view depicting diagrammatically the organization of one white pulp area. The periarteriolar sheath around the central arteriole is a thymus-dependent area (containing T-lymphocytes). The lymphatic follicles house cells of the B-series. The follicles frequently show germinal centres which have a lymphocytic "cap" rich in dendritic reticular cells. There may be one or more than one of these follicles per white pulp area. Peripherally there is a marginal sinus surrounded by a marginal zone.

1.8.4. *Functions of B-cells and T-cells*

The effector cells of the B-lineage secrete antibody. Any one cell is restricted not only in its combining specificity, but probably also in other characteristics of the immunoglobulin which it produces, such as the class and the light chain type. In the T-lineage lymphocytes are the effector cells (figure 1.14). There are a number of different T-cell functions, and again it is likely that any one cell is limited in its potential role. These activities of T-cells include:

(i) Responses to histocompatibility antigens, *in vivo* as in allograft reactions and *in vitro* as in mixed lymphocyte cultures. In mixed

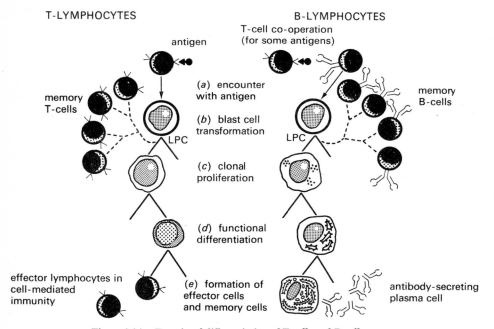

Figure 1.14. Functional differentiation of T-cells and B-cells
In both lines of immunocompetent cells (T-cells and B-cells), stimulation of a lymphocyte by antigen is followed first by blast cell transformation (with enlargement of the lymphocyte to form a large pyroninophilic cell (LPC)), then by a series of mitotic divisions which produce (i) effector cells of the immune system and (ii) sensitized lymphocytes which form memory cells. In the T-cell series the effector cells are lymphocytes (left of diagram). In the B-lineage they are plasma cells, formed by the acquisition of organelles (polyribosomes (represented as dots), endoplasmic reticulum and Golgi apparatus) as shown on the right of the diagram.

26 THE IMMUNE SYSTEM

lymphocyte cultures, the immunologically competent lymphocytes from one individual respond to histocompatibility antigens on the lymphocytes from the other by enlargement and then mitosis; experimentally these events can be followed by measuring the accompanying DNA synthesis. There is little or no memory component in mixed lymphocyte reactions, and pre-immunization is unnecessary.

(ii) T-cells from a specifically sensitized individual can act as killer lymphocytes and directly destroy any target cells in close proximity which bear the antigen against which the sensitivity was induced.

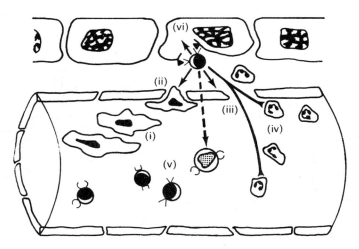

Figure 1.15. Soluble products of activated lymphocytes (lymphokine factors)

Some of the biological activities of the non-immunoglobulin factors (lymphokines) which are present in supernatant fluids recovered after stimulating sensitized lymphocytes with antigen are illustrated. These include:

(i) A chemotactic (chemically attracting) factor for macrophages.

(ii) A macrophage migration inhibition factor, MIF. ("In vivo" the chemotactic factor possibly attracts macrophages to the area of an immune reaction, and MIF keeps them there and probably activates them.)

(iii) A factor which increases vascular permeability.

(iv) A chemotactic factor for polymorph neutrophils (small phagocytes).

(v) A mitogenic factor which non-specifically evokes blastogenesis and proliferation of normal unsensitized lymphocytes.

(vi) A cytotoxic factor (lymphotoxin) which can kill various nucleated cells.

(iii) When sensitized T-lymphocytes are stimulated, they may liberate non-immunoglobulin agents (lymphokine factors). These are released specifically (in response to specific antigen) but they affect the activities of other cells in a non-specific way. Their actions may be due to a single substance or to several different substances, possibly produced by different cells. They include the inhibition of macrophage migration, effects on permeability, chemotactic attraction of monocytes (blood macrophages), and mitogenic effects (see figure 1.15). The non-specific anti-viral agent, interferon, may well belong to this group of lymphokine factors. It is also probable that soluble substances specifically released from T-cells are responsible for the type of cell-mediated immunity that occurs in infections of the tuberculosis type, and that a lymphokine (possibly the macrophage

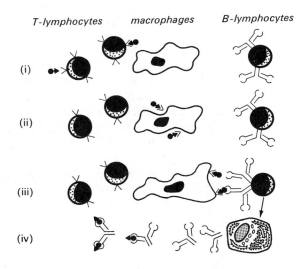

Figure 1.16.   Cellular co-operation in antibody production
Several models have been proposed to explain how T-cells help B-cells in the induction of antibody formation. This diagram outlines one possible mechanism. In this scheme: (i) A specific T-cell recognizes an antigenic determinant on the antigen (the carrier determinant, represented by a triangle). (ii) The T-cell releases an antigen-specific factor, a complex which binds to the surface of a macrophage and (iii) presents another determinant (the hapten, represented by a circle) in such a way that it stimulates a hapten-specific B-cell to differentiate towards effector function. (iv) The resulting plasma cell produces specific anti-hapten antibody. In the more general sense, each determinant on an antigen may be regarded as a hapten with the remainder of the molecule acting as a carrier.

migration inhibition factor) is responsible for bestowing upon macrophages the ability to kill organisms within their cytoplasm. Although specifically released from T-cells, this factor is non-specific in its action, and enables macrophages to kill any organism which they have phagocytosed.

(iv) T-cells have a role in regulating the production of antibody by B-cells. This role may be suppressive, and T-cells may contribute to part of the feed-back mechanisms which bring antibody production to an end. Perhaps even more important is their positive role in helping B-cells to become stimulated. These "helper cells" are necessary for antibody production to many antigens, although they do not themselves produce antibody. Their exact role in enabling B-cells to do so is uncertain, but it appears to involve mechanisms for effective presentation of the antigen to the B-cell. Since most antigenic molecules are mosaics of different antigenic determinants, the T-cells probably recognize some of these (the "carrier determinants"), combine with them, and perhaps liberate a complex which binds to the surface of a macrophage and presents another determinant (the hapten) in such a way that it stimulates the B-cell (figure 1.16). This probably involves a multiple presentation or concentration of the hapten determinant, since the few antigens which can stimulate B-cells without the help of T-cells are polymeric forms, i.e. they have repeating identical determinants, e.g. pneumococcal polysaccharide. It seems that physical contact between T-cells and B-cells is not essential for co-operation. Soluble factors are probably involved; these include an antigen-specific agent which acts at the stage of presentation, and a non-specific mitogenic factor which helps to expand the B-cell clone.

1.9. Comparative studies

Immune systems can be categorized and assessed as follows:

(i) Specific recognition: the occurrence of histoincompatibility phenomena; the scope of antigens recognized and the degree of discrimination.

(ii) Cell-mediated and humoral immune responses: the spectrum of available effector mechanisms, their kinetics and strength.

(iii) Immunological memory: its occurrence, duration and intensity.

(iv) Interdependence of the specific and non-specific components of the defence mechanisms.

(v) Structure and function of the lymphoid system: cell and tissue specializations; heterogeneity of cellular populations.

These criteria provide useful guidelines for our comparative studies.

CHAPTER TWO

INVERTEBRATE DEFENCE MECHANISMS

POSSESSION OF AN IMMUNE SYSTEM, ENCOMPASSING SPECIFIC IMMUNOLOGICAL recognition and memory with cell-mediated and humoral immune reactions, was until the 1970s popularly considered to be the exclusive property of vertebrates: invertebrate defence systems relied upon phagocytosis and showed only a crude specificity. These beliefs were bolstered by reports (see Chapter 3) that not even all the vertebrates possessed an immune potential.

In the present chapter we shall examine evidence for the existence of immunological reactivity at the various levels of invertebrate phylogeny. The subject is, however, in its infancy and many gaps remain. Also, in tracing the evolutionary development of the immune response, we are relying entirely on present-day species, an important point to bear in mind, particularly where the invertebrates are concerned: this group consists of several phyla, whereas vertebrates represent just one subphylum within a single phylum. A great variety in invertebrate defence mechanisms is therefore to be anticipated; equally, similarities between phyla are likely to be of fundamental significance.

2.1. Protozoa

Incompatibilities

A nucleus of one strain of amoeba may be transplanted to an enucleated "syngeneic" strain and the recipient will survive, whereas with nuclei from disparate strains, the greater the disparity, the less chance the recipient has for survival. However, unlike metazoan transplantation reactions which are mediated at cell surfaces, this protozoan incompatibility is intracellular and enzymatic rather than immunological.

In other experiments, if pieces of pseudopodia from amoeboid protozoa (*Difflugia*, *Arcella*) are separated by up to 500 μm from the mother cell, fragment and mother cell move towards each other and fuse. Fragments also fuse with pseudopodia of sister cells, but never with cells of another species. Here, although cell surfaces are involved, the actual means of recognition may be quite different from recognition in the immunological sense (i.e. by specific membrane-borne receptors: see section 1.3), since two lines from the same race grown in different media soon become incompatible, and compatibility is regained if they are grown again in the same medium.

Phagocytosis

The phagocytic system provides the most obvious link between the protozoa and metazoa. This system involving engulfment and subsequent digestion of particulate material has been utilized for a variety of functions, including feeding, removal of debris, and defence against infection. Though the relative significance of these functions differs at different phylogenetic levels, phagocytosis has remained essentially the same from protozoa through to the most advanced vertebrates. Again, some means of recognizing self versus non-self must be involved.

2.2. Simple metazoa

2.2.1. Sponges

Tissue incompatibilities

"Like" colonies of sponges will fuse together, "unlike" will not. Similarly, when sponges of two different species are disaggregated, and the cell suspensions from the two species are then mixed, each single aggregate that results appears to be composed of the cells of one of the species alone, although temporary aggregation of cells from different species may occur. The aggregation has been attributed to a large glycoprotein molecule (90S) which is heat-labile and which may be released intact by exposure of cells to calcium- and magnesium-free water. In some combinations, glycoprotein from one species has no effect on aggregation of cells from a second species, but this is not so for all species combinations. Species-specific adherence of sponge cells appears to be similar to tissue-specific cell aggregation in higher animals, but the molecular basis of the specificity is a matter of debate. Species incompatibility in sponges does not involve any cell damage or killing.

Phagocytosis and encapsulation

The phenomenon of phagocytosis is augmented in sponges and other metazoa by encapsulation: particles not dealt with readily by engulfment are instead "walled-off" by amoeboid cells (amoebocytes). In sponges (and in invertebrates in general), phagocytosis and encapsulation together provide a highly efficient means of body defence. In the marine sponge *Terpios*, for example, human erythrocytes injected into the mesogloea were encapsulated or phagocytosed, and then removed from the body by migration of the erythrocyte-enveloping or erthyrocyte-laden cells into excurrent canals, all within 48 hours (at 22 °C). In these "lowly" metazoa, the amoebocytes concerned are free-wandering cells occurring scattered in the mesogloea: there is no organization of defensive cells into tissues.

2.2.2. Coelenterates

Tissue incompatibilities

Although primitive in organization (e.g. in the lack of blood-vascular and organ systems), coelenterates are not only able to discriminate between self and non-self but may even show quasi-immune reactions, leading to death of non-syngeneic cells. Recent studies on hard corals (*Acropora*), for example, have shown that if the soft tissues of intra-colony branches are joined, they will eventually fuse; joining of inter-colony branches of the same species eventually leads to tissue destruction in the contact zone; and joining of inter-colony branches of different species also leads to cell destruction, but more rapidly (in approximately one week at 25 °C). The mechanism of killing is not clear, but the fact that there is a period of fusion before tissue destruction occurs suggests that it is not due to straightforward anatomical or biochemical incompatibilities.

Somewhat similar incompatibilities have been observed in other coelenterates. In the colonial hydroid *Hydractinia*, clones derived asexually from single colonies fuse compatibly; unrelated (allogeneic) colonies consistently fail to fuse when in contact. In this case, hyperplastic growth of stolons of one or both strains occurs in the area of contact, followed by regression of the strain with lesser hyperplastic potential. In gorgonian corals, autografts survive indefinitely, but allografts and xenografts are rejected. In incompatible combinations, tissue destruction occurs only in the smaller colony. Studies using antimetabolites have suggested that one strain does not itself kill the second, but instead triggers off a "suicide" mechanism. In *Hydra*, a solitary fresh-water coelenterate, orthotopic allografts (i.e. grafts placed in a position similar to that from which they derived) are usually accepted, even though hydra pairs which are found to be compatible do not have in common all the potentially antigenic macromolecules which can be identified by immunoelectrophoresis. However, eventual separation has been reported following grafting between *Hydra viridis* isolated from different ponds. *Hydra* xenografts do not survive permanently, although persistence may be prolonged. Migratory interstitial cells have been found in xenografts, but there is no direct evidence that they are responsible for rejection. Moreover, no memory component has been established in any of these coelenterate reactions.

Phagocytosis

As in sponges, the coelenterate mesogloea may contain wandering amoebocytes. There is no organization of these phagocytes into distinct tissues.

2.3. Protostomes

On the basis of embryological evidence, and to a lesser extent on skeletal arrangement and difference in phosphagens, the bilateral Metazoa have been separated into two superphyla, the Protostomia (embracing annelids, molluscs and arthropods) and Deuterostomia (including the echinoderms and chordates). This classification is a useful one in emphasizing two main evolutionary streams within the invertebrates (see figure 2.1) and in pointing to affinities between vertebrates and the deuterostome invertebrates. The protostomes are by far the most important invertebrate group in terms of the number of species they represent, but they and the deuterostomes have gone their separate ways since Precambrian times, both superphyla being already well established in the Cambrian fauna of 500 million years ago.

2.3.1. *Platyhelminthes*

The deuterostomes appear to have diverged from the protostome line at a point beyond the Platyhelminthes (flatworms), but the latter are included here under the protostome "umbrella": although acoelomate, they show similar embryology to annelids and molluscs.

Transplantation reactions

Little is known of possible specific immune reactions in flatworms. Transplantation experiments on various regions of planarians were undertaken, especially in the early 1930s, but these were designed to investigate the control of morphogenesis rather than immunological phenomena. Grafts were often successful, even between different species, but whether this is attributable to absence of immune potential, a tolerance effect, or inappropriate experimental conditions, cannot be decided on available evidence.

Phagocytosis

Carbon particles entering the skin of experimentally wounded trematodes (*Haematoloechus* and *Megalodiscus*) are engulfed by a population of

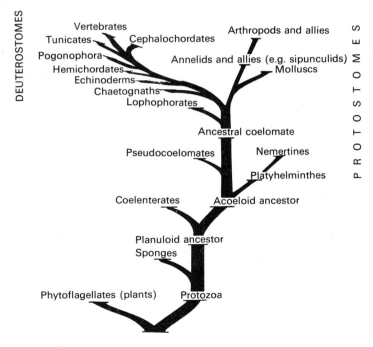

Figure 2.1. Phylogenetic relationships in the animal kingdom
Partly from Barnes, R. D. (1963), *Invertebrate Zoology*, W. B. Saunders & Co. Ltd. Philadelphia (with modifications).

phagocytes in the parenchymatous tissue. These then apparently migrate into the intestinal caeca and are eliminated from the body via the mouth (there is no anal exit at this phylogenetic level). Such a mechanism may also be responsible for the removal of pathogenic organisms.

2.3.2. Nemertines

Nemertines closely resemble the platyhelminthes in their general organization. They are, however, the most primitive invertebrates to possess a true circulatory system. Amoeboid cells derived from yolk-filled cells have been observed in the circulation.

Transplantation reactions

Recent orthotopic grafting experiments made on species of *Lineus* (Heteronemertina) have shown that in all cases allografts are accepted, and they retain their own pigmentation. Given consistent experimental parameters, the xenograft reaction can take one of three forms, depending on the inter-specific combination used: there may be survival of all grafts; rapid rejection of all grafts; or survival or rejection according to the individual. The rejection process consists of depigmentation and marginal resorption, followed by expulsion of the central necrotic region by the graft recipient. It seems likely that nemertines are able to respond to certain xenogeneic tissues by an immunological means. Where first-set (i.e. first-time) xenografts are rejected, an accelerated second-set rejection has been demonstrated; this indicates a memory component, though the degree of specificity of this has not been established.

2.3.3. Annelids

Transplantation reactions

Extensive studies by independent groups of workers have demonstrated specific skin transplantation immunity and memory in annelids. The speed of rejection is directly related to temperature. At 15 °C, first-set xenografts exchanged between earthworms of the genera *Lumbricus* and *Eisenia* (see figure 2.2) are destroyed at times between 8 and 147 days (usually approximately 30 days, in either direction of the exchange, the end-point being determined by pigment cell destruction). Second-set xenografts are destroyed either more quickly (positive memory) or more slowly (negative memory) at this temperature. For reasons not yet understood, increasing the reaction temperature (to 20 °C) tips the balance towards positive rather than negative memory. The memory is specific: rejection times of grafts from a third party (e.g. grafts from earthworms of the genus *Allolobophora*) placed on *Lumbricus* do not affect, and are not affected by, the *Lumbricus* anti-*Eisenia* reaction times.

Unlike nemertines, where only xenograft rejection has been demonstrated, annelids are also able to reject allografts. However, the reaction is weak and slow (38–153 days in *Lumbricus*, 15–255 days in *Eisenia*, at 15 °C), even where animals from remote localities are used. As in xenograft rejection, rejection of second-set allografts may be prolonged or curtailed. This phenomenon, wherein the repeat graft may elicit either positive or negative memory, has also been described in vertebrates (see, for example, section 5.1.1).

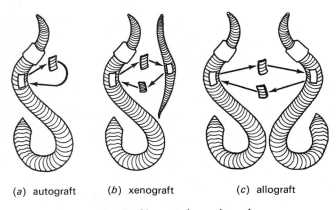

(*a*) autograft   (*b*) xenograft   (*c*) allograft

Figure 2.2.   Grafting experiments in earthworms

(*a*) Autografts of an animal's own tissues, depicted here in the earthworm *Lumbricus*, heal promptly and show no signs of rejection.

(*b*) Xenografts exchanged between animals of different species (e.g. *Lumbricus* and *Eisenia*) heal at first but are always eventually destroyed.

(*c*) Allografts made between individuals of the same species (e.g. in *Lumbricus terrestris*) are also rejected, but in earthworms the alloimmune response is weak and slow.

After Cooper, E. L. (1968), "Transplantation Immunity in Annelids. 1. Rejection of Xenografts exchanged between *Lumbricus terrestris* and *Eisenia foetida*", *Transplantation*, **6**, 322–337, and Cooper, E. L. (1969), "Chronic Allograft Rejection in *Lumbricus terrestris*", *Journal of Experimental Zoology*, **171**, 69–74.

Interesting parallels between earthworm graft rejection and that in more advanced animals are also seen at the cellular level: rejection involves invasion of the graft by cells (coelomocytes), and these can transfer anti-xenograft immunity to a non-immune worm. In addition, increased numbers of coelomocytes are associated with second-set grafts compared with first-set grafts, thus providing a cellular basis for the gross manifestations of memory. The proposed sequence of events is illustrated in figure 2.3.

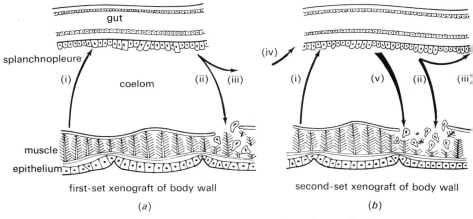

first-set xenograft of body wall
(a)

second-set xenograft of body wall
(b)

Figure 2.3. Xenograft rejection in the earthworm *Eisenia*

(a) First-set graft. Antigenic stimulation from the xenograft induces proliferation in small undifferentiated cells of the coelomic lining (splanchnopleure cells) with the production of coelomocytes, mainly macrophages (i). These attack the graft (ii) and also migrate to other parts of the body (iii).

(b) Second-set graft. A second xenograft from the same species also elicits responses (i), (ii) and (iii). In addition, sensitized cells resulting from the first exposure to antigenic stimulation (iv) quickly attack the graft (v). The second-set xenograft reaction therefore occurs more rapidly and is more intense than the first-set response.

From Valembois, P. (1971), "Rôle des leucocytes dans l'acquisition d'une immunité antigreffe spécifique chez les Lombriciens", *Archives de Zoologie expérimentale et générale*, **112**, 97–103 (with modifications).

The coelomocytes implicated are phagocytic, with an eccentric nucleus, and belong to a family of cells derived from the splanchnopleure. Like the lymphocytes of vertebrates, they respond to non-specific mitogens (phytohaemagglutinin (PHA) and concanavalin A), but attempts to produce a reaction in "mixed lymphocyte cultures" have not yet been successful.

Humoral factors

Although annelids clearly show cell-mediated immune reactions, no antibodies (immunoglobulins) are present. However, the coelomic fluid of some earthworms (e.g. *Eisenia*), like the serum of some amphibians, contains a cytolytic factor (lipoprotein or lipoprotein-bound) which non-specifically lyses various vertebrate erythrocytes. These lysins are synthesized by free chloragocytes in the coelomic fluid.

Phagocytosis and encapsulation

Earthworm coelomocytes (amoebocytes) play an important role in phago-cytosing foreign particles and bacteria, and they seem to be capable of discrimination in relation to materials injected into the coelomic cavity. For example, mammalian sperm or sperm from a worm of a different species are phagocytosed after an interval of about 20 hours, but allogeneic sperm are not. Carbon and carmine particles and a variety of bacteria are engulfed more rapidly than foreign sperms or erythrocytes. The lining cells of the coelom, through active proliferation, rapidly renew the supply of coelomocytes.

Large invaders such as nematode parasites evoke an encapsulation response in worms. This involves invasion of the area by amoebocytes and formation of a fibrous capsule (which eventually becomes calcified) surrounding the parasite.

"Lymphoid tissues"

Unlike the scattered amoeboid cells of the simple invertebrates, such as the sponges and coelenterates, discrete foci can be identified in annelids. The dorsal blood vessel of earthworms and leeches, for example, has "valves" which are primarily sites of budding amoeboid cells, and only secondarily perform a mechanical function in the circulation. Similarly, haemal glands adhering to this blood vessel in the midgut region of earth-worms populate the coelomic fluid and blood with red cells, phagocytes and non-phagocytic granulocytes. Such aggregations in earthworms have often been described in vertebrate terminology (e.g. "lymphoid tissues", "lymph glands"), but it seems premature to assume homologies regarding the tissues themselves or their cellular products.

2.3.4. *Sipunculids*

Sipunculids are coelomate marine worms related to the annelids.

Humoral factors

In the sipunculid worm *Dendrostomum*, a circulating humoral factor with bactericidal (cytotoxic) activity has been induced following immunization with a Gram-negative bacillus. In non-immunized worms and most worms examined 1–7 days after immunization, no bactericidins were detected in the coelomic fluid, but at 60 days after stimulation, positive results were obtained. A repeated injection of bacteria on day 60 elicited significantly enhanced bactericidin titres. The degree of specificity of this reaction was not determined, but in another sipunculid species, a factor which caused lysis of a parasitic marine ciliate could be induced by injection of crab blood with or without the ciliate, or by injecting large numbers of bacteria. Thus inducible humoral responses can be readily demonstrated in sipunculids, but their specificity is not comparable with that of the immune response of vertebrates.

Urn cells and phagocytes

The sipunculid coelomic fluid contains a great variety of free cells, including red blood cells, phagocytic amoebocytes, granulocytes, and the remarkable mucus-secreting urn cells. This mucus is secreted as a consequence of infection, and only foreign cells stick to it: "self" cells do not. Also, different kinds of mucus are secreted which recognize different foreign cells. Particulate matter trapped in the mucus is then engulfed by phagocytes. We have, therefore, a refinement of recognition in sipunculids, together with specialization of phagocytes, involving cooperation with a second cell type and/or humoral factors.

Encapsulation

Dendrostomum recognizes implanted foreign, damaged or stained eggs, and reacts by encapsulating them with amoebocytes, but it does not treat its own intact eggs as foreign when these are implanted.

2.3.5. *Molluscs*

Transplantation reactions

Work on transplantation in molluscs has suffered from technical difficulties, and little decisive evidence is available. The animals are often unable to withstand repeated grafting and prolonged observation at elevated temperatures; mucous coats may interfere with the reaction; few molluscan tissues are very distinctive; improved ways of measuring normal physiological function of the transplanted tissues are needed; and unfortunately experiments which have been carried out so far have often employed heterotopic ("unnaturally" located) grafts rather than orthotopic grafts. It is reported that autografts, allografts and xenografts can be distinguished—host cell reactions of snails to xenogeneic tissue occur more rapidly and are more severe than those involving allografts—but precise estimations of specificity and memory are lacking.

Humoral factors

This, by contrast, is a well-studied field, particularly in commercially or medically important molluscan species. In snails (*Helix*), for example, haemagglutinins are found in the albumin gland which define antigens in the ABO and some MN systems of human erythrocytes. They can distinguish between different carbohydrate groups, and provide highly specific stable reagents for detecting carbohydrate receptors of normal and neoplastic blood and tissue cell surfaces. These snail haemagglutinins are protein and multivalent and have disulphide bonds, but they are not immunoglobulins. They do, however, constitute a defence system in the snail, since they agglutinate bacteria and bind larval parasites; they have been found not only in the albumin glands, where they are involved in protecting the eggs, but also in the eggs themselves when examined two weeks after their deposition in the environment, and in adult haemolymph. It is worth noting here that antibody-like substances can also be demonstrated in fish roe. It is also of interest that snails of the same species from different geographical regions show different reactions of their agglutinins, also that agglutinins from the albumin gland are different from those in the haemolymph.

Natural haemagglutinins with varying degrees of specificity for diverse foreign erythrocytes have been described in the body fluids of several other gastropods and a bivalve (oyster). They are all proteins or have a protein component, but molecular weights are variable: oyster haemagglutinin is mainly 34S with some 29S and 13S; *Aplysia* (sea hare) agglutinating activity is due to a heterogeneous group of molecules ranging from approximately 18·5S to 31S. Unlike vertebrate antibodies, none are specifically inducible by immunization, although it is claimed that some invertebrate haemagglutinins, e.g. in the oyster, have small subunits of molecular weight similar to the light chains (L chains) of vertebrate immunoglobulins. Inducible bactericidins can be demonstrated in several species of abalone (*Haliotis*), but their appearance, unlike that of antibody, is rapid and transient, peaking at 1–2 days.

Phagocytosis and encapsulation

Oysters readily phagocytose injected carbon particles and erythrocytes, bacteria, bacterial spores and yeast. Tissues are cleared by phagocytes (amoebocytes) carrying ingested particles through epithelia to the exterior, or by intracellular digestion. Molluscs also encapsulate many kinds of foreign materials in their tissues: planorbid snails, for example, are able to encapsulate—and therefore isolate—eggs and larvae of parasites, pollen, certain bacteria, and implanted tissues.

Opsonization

It appears that the main defence mechanism of molluscs depends on subtle interactions between phagocytes and humoral factors in the haemolymph. In the octopus *Eledone*, phagocytosis is dependent on the presence of octopus humoral factors; the phagocytes of some other molluscs can act without haemolymph, but their capabilities are enhanced in its presence. There is thus good evidence of opsonization in invertebrates. The source and mechanisms of the factors involved are little understood, although it is known that some opsonins are also haemagglutinins.

Antigen clearance

Immunocompetence in vertebrates is often demonstrated by specifically accelerated clearance of an antigen from the circulation following a repeated injection. This increased rate of clearance is associated with elevation of antibody titre. Secondary clearance can also be demonstrated in some molluscs (e.g. oysters, *Crassostrea* and sea hares, *Aplysia*) and arthropods (e.g. crabs, *Carcinus*, see section 2.3.6), although it could not be demonstrated in a sipunculid. The oyster can clear a secondary injection of T2 bacteriophage more rapidly than a primary one, but the response is not entirely specific; animals given a primary injection with an unrelated bacteriophage and then challenged later with T2 still showed accelerated elimination of T2, albeit less rapid than when T2 was also the primary stimulus. The effect seems to have a cellular basis in the oyster, since a prolonged schedule of immunization with T2 did not elicit circulating "antibody".

"Lymphoid tissues"

The evolutionary trend of phagocytes and other cells associated with the circulation to form into tissues, as we have described in the annelids (section 2.3.3), is seen even more clearly in molluscs, particularly in cephalopods such as the octopus: these have distinct haemopoietic centres in the form of "white bodies" and "branchial spleens", together with a sophisticated vascular system; phagocytosis in the octopus *Eledone* occurs localized in the haemopoietic organs, gills, salivary glands and blood. In the gastropod *Aplysia* (sea hare), a large concentration of haemocytes at the base of the gill filaments has been described, similar histologically to octopus "white bodies"; this is also a site of phagocytosis.

2.3.6. Arthropods

Transplantation reactions and encapsulation

Most experiments to date suggest that arthropods fail to recognize allografts and even some xenografts as foreign. However, genetic or embryological, rather than immunological, questions have provided much of the stimulus for work in this field, and critical evidence is surprisingly limited.

Among cockroaches (*Periplaneta*), skin transplanted between nymphs, or from adult to nymphs, retains its integrity through successive moults. Similarly, orthotopic allografts of legs between adult crayfish (*Cambarus*) remain viable for many weeks at 25 °C, even after moulting. Where rejections have been observed, an encapsulation reaction is employed. Adult cockroaches (*Leucophaea*), for example, destroy diverse vertebrate cell lines of normal or neoplastic origin by accumulating haemocytes around the transplanted cell clusters, leading to encapsulation and necrosis. This procedure does not appear to have a memory component, since a second exposure to the same line of culture cells neither accelerated nor prolonged the response. Nevertheless, encapsulation in insects may involve a discrimination beyond that of self versus non-self, namely, between different types of non-self. Thus insect larvae (*Pimpla*), injected with allogeneic or xenogeneic eggs will encapsulate xenogeneic eggs to a greater degree (by forming a thicker cellular capsule) than allogeneic ones.

Phagocytosis

Insect haemocytes are able to engulf colloidal substances, ink and carmine particles, bacteria, fungi, protozoa and vertebrate erythrocytes. Although the efficiency of the process can vary greatly, depending on the nature and the amount of the substance introduced, species, stage and physiological condition of the host and environmental temperature, it is nonetheless clear that phagocytosis and encapsulation are major components of the arthropod defence system.

Humoral factors

Humoral factors, as in molluscs, are fairly well studied in arthropods, particularly in those species which are of commercial importance. Lobsters (*Homarus americanus*), for example, are known to possess naturally occurring haemagglutinins which are capable of opsonization. Thus, under *in vitro* conditions, human erythrocytes are poorly encapsulated or phagocytosed by washed haemocytes, but with agglutinins added, the erythrocytes are dealt with efficiently. Lobster haemagglutinins appear to derive from haemocytes, since haemagglutinating activity in haemocyte extracts is about 100 times greater than for haemocyte-free haemolymph, and the number of haemocytes contributing to the extract is proportional to the titre obtained. In addition, agglutinin titres in normal haemolymph can be related to total haemocyte counts.

As in molluscs, some crustacean haemagglutinins are highly specific, others will cross-react with a variety of foreign erythrocytes. They appear to be proteins (11S and more than 19S in lobsters) but are not inducible. It has been reported in crabs, as in oysters, that the haemagglutinin contains small subunits of molecular weight similar to vertebrate light chains (L chains), though structural homologies between vertebrate and invertebrate haemagglutinins are usually denied.

Bactericidal substances can be induced in lobsters as in certain molluscan and sipunculid species. Haemolymph from spiny lobsters (*Panulirus*) tested against EMB-1, a Gram-negative enteric bacillus, showed little or no natural (i.e. pre-existing) levels of bactericidin, but these appeared after a primary injection of bacteria, with titres peaking at 1–2 days; live cultures or killed vaccines proved equally effective. Variable results were obtained when titres were tested against bacteria other than EMB-1. Enhanced responses—an even more rapid appearance and longer peak titres—were demonstrated following secondary injection of bacteria. This humoral response in *Panulirus* therefore has a memory component, but it lacks the specificity of the vertebrate antibody response, and appears much more rapidly. This lobster bactericidin is of high molecular weight, but its chemical nature is obscure. A similar rapid bactericidal response has also been induced in the lobster *Homarus* following injection with *Pseudomonas perolens* vaccine, with an 8-fold increase in titre appearing 2 days after stimulation. Natural haemagglutinin titres determined for the same haemolymph samples during this period were unaffected by the bactericidal response.

Injection of bacteria into insects, e.g. wax moth (*Galleria*) larvae and milkweed bugs (*Oncopeltus*), again induces a rapid bactericidal response, peaking at 24 hours after injection. Sites of the response in wax moth larvae appear to be located throughout the body. It is reported that these insect bactericidins are non-protein in nature, but the chemical basis of bactericidal activity in arthropods, and in invertebrates in general, is very much at issue. Precipitins have also been detected in the circulation of some insects and lobsters, but they are unlike vertebrate precipitins and do not appear to be common.

Antigen clearance

The crab *Carcinus* is able to eliminate T1 bacteriophage from its circulation two or three times as rapidly on rechallenge as compared with a single injection of T1. Although no control specificity tests were reported, these results suggest a memory component in the crab. The memory appears to have a cellular rather than humoral basis, since no neutralizing activity against T1 could be detected in the haemolymph. This phenomenon resembles that seen in oysters (section 2.3.5).

Studies on snails (*Helix*) and crayfish (*Parachaeraps*) comparing clearance of carbon (non-antigenic particles) from the circulation have shown that both in crustaceans and in molluscs there is a highly active system of phagocytes, mainly associated with the liver-like digestive diverticula. Even though its phagocytic system is less widespread than that of the snail, the crayfish showed the more rapid clearance of particles from its circulation (at room temperature), possibly due to a more rapid vascular transport and therefore increased chance of contact between particles and phagocytes.

"Lymphoid tissues"

The origins of the circulating cells (haemocytes) in insect haemolymph have been a matter of controversy for some time. Distinct haemopoietic tissues have, however, been identified in *Locusta, Gryllus, Calliphora* and *Melolontha*; and in *Locusta* it has been shown that X-irradiation of the haemopoietic organ (situated in the dorsal region adjacent to the haemocoel) brings about a marked decrease in the animal's haemocyte count. The same organ is also concerned with phagocytosis of debris from the circulation.

Following immunization of *Locusta* with live bacteria (*Bacillus thuringiensis*), two types of reaction are evident in the haemopoietic tissue: (i) intense proliferation of reticular cells possessing phagocytic and haemopoietic potentialities, with the liberation of numerous young cells into the haemolymph; (ii) differentiation of reticular cells into cells of a secretory type. This latter reaction correlates with the demonstration in *Locusta* haemolymph of soluble antibacterial factors and antitoxins (the nature and specificity of which are not yet clear). Reaction (ii) is the only one evident in reticular cells if bacterial toxin is injected instead of bacterial cells. This insect haemopoietic tissue, with its well-defined reactions to particulate and soluble antigens, and its important role in the renewal of haemocytes, is remarkably similar to vertebrate haemopoietic tissue, particularly when we take into account the evolutionary gulf which separates the two groups (figure 2.1).

2.4. Deuterostomes

In attempting to unravel the evolutionary sequence of events that culminated in the highly sophisticated immune system of vertebrates, a detailed scrutiny of the immune mechanisms in deuterostome invertebrates should be particularly fruitful, since it is from this line that the vertebrates themselves arose.

2.4.1. *Echinoderms*

Transplantation reactions

Under optimal conditions, namely orthotopic transplantation of clearly defined tissue and maintenance of experimental animals at reasonably high temperature over a prolonged period of time, echinoderms show unequivocal evidence of specific allograft immunity with at least short-term memory. Allogeneic incompatibility has been demonstrated in two sea stars *Protoreaster nodosus* and *Dermasterias imbricata*, and in the sea cucumber *Cucumaria tricolor*. Although initial (first-set) grafts in echino-

°derms persist for months before finally being rejected, repeat grafting of tissue from the same donor leads to progressively more rapid rejection. This memory is specific, since rejection of grafts from an unrelated donor is not accelerated. Echinoderm allografts undergoing rejection are infiltrated by coelomocytes of multiple types, including those resembling vertebrate macrophages, eosinophilic granulocytes and small lymphocytes; hyperplasia occurs along the contact zone, donor pigment cells are destroyed, and there is an invasive replacement of graft tissue. The role of each infiltrating cell type is unknown, but the gross and histological similarities between these echinoderm reactions and vertebrate allograft immunity are noteworthy. The major limitation of the transplantation reaction in echinoderms may prove to be in the short-term nature of its memory component.

Studies on starfish (*Asterias*) which have been inoculated with various cell preparations, both of xenogeneic and of allogeneic origin, suggest that the two types of antigenic tissue are treated differently: xenogeneic, but not allogeneic, cells bring about a release by the host of a soluble factor which activates host cell (amoebocyte) aggregation and thereby traps the injected cells. In this connection, it is perhaps pertinent to recall that the rejection of xenogeneic grafts mediated by amoebocytes in earthworms (section 2.3.3) is more efficient than rejection of allografts.

Coelomocytes

Coelomocytes of at least four morphologically distinct types have been identified in sea urchins (*Strongylocentrotus*). These include phagocytic leucocytes (amoebocytes), vibratile cells, red spherule cells and colourless spherule cells, and there is evidence of a division of labour in their respective defensive functions. The phagocytic leucocyte is the cell type involved in cell aggregation, and this process secondarily traps other cell types. The flagellated vibratile cells appear to have a dual purpose in keeping coelomic fluid in motion and thereby limiting cell aggregation, and in releasing a mucoid substance which causes the coelomic fluid to gel in areas of invasion by foreign liquids and other foreign material, so preventing invasion of the entire coelom. These vibratile cells are reminiscent of sipunculid urn cells (section 2.3.4). Spherule cell functions are obscure, but they may include formation of the collagenous material used in tissue repair.

It has been suggested that sea urchin coelomocytes—like vertebrate lymphocytes—possess receptor molecules which combine selectively with foreign proteins, since exposure of coelomocytes *in vitro* to bovine serum albumin (BSA) inhibits their subsequent uptake of BSA but not of the closely related human serum albumin (HSA). This process may be comparable with specific immunological recognition in vertebrates, but so far in echinoderms the specific antigen-binding has not been correlated with any specific immune response to these proteins.

In vitro studies using a hanging-drop technique have shown that the usual reaction of coelomocytes to Gram-negative bacteria (the most common marine bacteria) is the formation of a wall-like clot which effectively limits bacteria to the original point of inoculation. Both non-aggregated and partially aggregated cells enter into wall formation. The leucocytes are the only active agents, but other cell types are caught and incorporated into the clot. Red spherule cells may migrate to the edges of a leucocyte clot facing the bacteria to form a dense red border, and are able to immobilize motile bacteria. When a concentrated clump of these Gram-negative bacteria is deposited within a group of coelomocytes, the bacteria may be encapsulated by the wall of leucocytes and accompanying red spherule cells. In contrast, Gram-positive bacteria—which are much less common in the marine environment—do not elicit encapsulation or "walling-off" responses in sea urchins; instead only a "low-key" phagocytic response is evoked, similar to that elicited by non-antigenic particles such as carbon or latex. Echinoderm responses to different bacteria therefore show a graded recognition of non-self, but the processes of elimination are similar to those seen in invertebrates which are less close to the vertebrate stock.

Echinoderm humoral factors are poorly studied. Natural haemag-glutinins have been noted in holothuroid (sea cucumber) and asteroid (starfish and sea star) species, and there may be inducible factors, but there is as yet no evidence of an immunoglobulin-type molecule at this level of phylogeny. There are no discrete lymphoid (or lymphoid-like) organs as seen in vertebrates or in advanced protostomes.

2.4.2. *Tunicates*

Adult tunicates little resemble other chordates, but their larvae are considered to exhibit many of the features characteristic of the forerunners of the early vertebrates; indeed, it is thought by some authorities that the vertebrate stock derives from a larval tunicate ancestry by a process involving paedogenesis (retention of larval characters by the adult).

Transplantation and histocompatibility reactions

Extensive studies indicate the presence in tunicates of cells morphologically resembling vertebrate lymphocytes. In *Perophora* these cells, like vertebrate lymphocytes, are known to be sensitive to X-irradiation. Seven other distinct blood-cell types, including phagocytes, have been identified in this group.

Recent experiments on the solitary tunicate *Ciona* have shown that, while autografts are accepted, orthotopic allografts are rejected, and that the rejection is associated with an increase in lymphocytes and phagocytes. Investigations of a possible memory component in *Ciona* have so far been thwarted by difficulties in maintaining the experimental animals for

Table 2.1. Incompatibility reactions in tunicates and vertebrates

A. Incompatibility reactions in the tunicate *Botryllus primigenus*

Parents: AB × CD

F₁ Progeny

		AC	AD	BC	BD
Incompatible	AC				+
reactions	AD			+	
with:	BC		+		
	BD	+			

Result: 75% compatible
25% incompatible

B. Vertebrate histocompatibility reactions for strong histocompatibility loci

Parents: AB × CD

F₁ Progeny

		AC	AD	BC	BD
Incompatible	AC		+	+	+
reactions	AD	+		+	+
with:	BC	+	+		+
	BD	+	+	+	

Result: 25% compatible
75% incompatible

prolonged periods of time in aquaria. *Ciona* lymphocytes, like vertebrate T-lymphocytes, proliferate in the presence of phytohaemagglutinin (PHA) and they respond to the presence of allogeneic lymphocytes in mixed lymphocyte cultures.

Allogeneic recognition is also seen in the colonial tunicates *Botryllus*, *Perophora* and *Amaroucium*. The tunic and vascular stolon of compatible colonies placed in contact fuse to form a continuous tube, allowing exchange of blood cells, nutrients, etc. Conversely, the tunic at the site of contact between incompatible colonies thickens without fusion, and a local necrosis may subsequently occur similar to that described in colonial coelenterates (section 2.2.2). Studies on *Botryllus primigenus* have attributed control of colony specificity to a single gene locus with multiple alleles, but the criteria for compatibility seem to be unlike those usually displayed by vertebrates. Thus, in the case shown in Table 2.1, there is a $3:1$ chance of compatibility between the F_1 progeny; individuals differing by a single haplotype (one allele of the pair) are compatible, whereas in vertebrates, a single haplotype difference for the major histocompatibility region usually leads to rejection. This may indicate a "set of rules" in tunicates which is different from that of vertebrates, and which involves positive recognition of the shared allele. On the other hand, there are circumstances in vertebrates where a gene dose effect is apparent, and a one-haplotype difference results in a weaker reaction than a two-haplotype difference. If this is the case in *Botryllus*, it may be that tolerance effects are operating in a system which is essentially similar to that of vertebrates.

Humoral factors

Natural non-inducible haemagglutinins have been described in tunicates, but vertebrate-type circulating antibodies appear to be absent. Cell-free and whole coelomic fluid of *Ciona* killed or depressed the numbers of obligately marine Gram-negative bacteria *in vitro* but did not affect a facultatively marine Gram-positive micrococcus or a Gram-negative terrestrial bacterium. The normal body fluids of *Ciona* thus appear to have their major inhibitory effect on the bacterial species the tunicate commonly encounters, though how the distinction is achieved is unclear.

Phagocytosis and encapsulation

If foreign erythrocytes are injected into the *Ciona* tunic, they are first agglutinated, but their subsequent fate depends on the dose injected: if few, the cells will be phagocytosed; if many, they will be encapsulated, then ejected from the body. A secondary injection of erythrocytes 6 days after the first can elicit an encapsulation response for doses which failed to elicit encapsulation after the first injection. There thus appears to be a memory component associated with this defence mechanism in *Ciona*. Specificity is lacking, however, since injection of duck erythrocytes following an injection of human erythrocytes still elicits a secondary response to the duck cells.

It is concluded that certain tunicate defence mechanisms that we have just described (e.g. the encapsulation phenomenon) are more closely allied to those of other invertebrates than to vertebrate reactions, whereas the blood cells and the transplantation responses of tunicates and vertebrates are closely comparable. Thus the immunological status of tunicates seems to reflect their unique evolutionary position.

2.5. Conclusions

An essential first step in maintaining the integrity of the body is the ability to distinguish between self and non-self, and this ability is present in all animal groups. However, as we have seen, recognition is involved with a broad spectrum of situations, not all of which—phagocytic nutrition and sponge cell aggregation, for example—form part of an immune response. Immunological recognition in vertebrates is apparently dependent on immunoglobulin placed in a membrane as a recognizing molecule, and this immunoglobulin molecule is regarded by many as the essence of immunology. Since no invertebrates are known to possess secreted immunoglobulins, does this mean that their cellular receptor sites are different from those of vertebrates? Clearly, we need more information on the degree of uniformity in the molecular mechanisms of cellular recognition, through the invertebrates to vertebrates, before we can decide on their affinities.

Invertebrate humoral factors as a whole present a bewildering picture. The haemagglutinins found in various invertebrates (including protostomes) appear to resemble vertebrate antibody (immunoglobulin), at least insofar as they are protein; they may have opsonizing properties and may show a high degree of specificity, but they are not inducible by immunization, and their molecular structures show little uniformity. The ability of these invertebrate proteins (like vertebrate antibodies) to bind selectively to specific carbohydrates forming cell surface receptors does, however, suggest an early evolutionary development of protein-carbohydrate recognition mechanisms. Inducible humoral factors (with bactericidal properties) do exist in invertebrates, but they are not completely specific and, like the agglutinins, are heterogeneous in their molecular structure. The question of phylogenetic relationships between immunoglobulin and non-immunoglobulin humoral factors is a fascinating but quite open one. The vertebrates do not appear to have abandoned these other factors once they acquired immunoglobulins: it has been established that some vertebrate factors with specific receptor sites for erythrocytes or certain polysaccharides have structures different from the known immunoglobulins.

Whilst the capacity to synthesize immunoglobulin molecules appears to be a property of the vertebrates alone, there is now good evidence that specific cell-mediated immunity (as shown by skin graft reactions) arose much earlier in evolution, and is already well established in the higher invertebrates. In echinoderms, for example, there is a sharp discrimination at the level of antigenic recognition, even though the rejection process is slow and the memory component may prove to be of limited duration. These cell-mediated reactions in deuterostome invertebrates are very similar to those in the vertebrates. Other skin graft reactions, notably in annelids, are more controversial: are they homologous with the vertebrate reactions—in which case specific cell-mediated immunity, with memory, must have evolved at a point earlier than that at which the protostomes and deuterostomes diverged—or do they represent a parallel evolution (analogy)? Perhaps we should again state the problem in terms of recognition mechanisms: to ask whether the foreign tissues placed on annelids and vertebrates are being recognized in a comparable way; whether there are similar surface receptors on vertebrate T-lymphocytes and earthworm coelomocytes. More information is needed, not only concerning the immunocompetent cells in invertebrates, but also on the nature of their histocompatibility antigens.

Despite the great diversity of types among invertebrates, the basic pattern of response to foreign matter (both living and dead) and to tissue injury, is remarkably constant. In general, amoeboid cells (amoebocytes) phagocytose small particles, while larger particles are encapsulated. Removal of offending material is generally highly efficient: substances not degraded within amoebocytes may be eliminated from the tissues as host amoebocytes migrate through the epithelial layers to the exterior. Why has a complex lymphoid system, such as we see in the vertebrates, become "superimposed" on their phagocytic system? It is possible that, in the vertebrates especially, progressive specialization of the tissues and their greater insulation from the environment have impaired the efficiency of the phagocytes in removing foreign organisms and created a need for additional forms of protection: unlike the rapid elimination of foreign particulate matter by most invertebrates, disposal in mammals is slow, except from the lungs, and injected particles may persist for many years. Alternatively, the lymphoid complex may have evolved to accentuate the fineness of discrimination. Discrimination in phagocytosis by mammals, and possibly by some of the higher invertebrates (e.g. molluscs and arthropods), is due predominantly to specific humoral factors (opsonins) acting as recognition factors. What may have begun as a mere facilitation of phagocytosis by non-specific factors in some ancestral invertebrate culminated in the largely serum-dependent mammalian system with its involvement of specific opsonic immunoglobulins.

It has been postulated that the fine discrimination afforded by the immune system (lymphoid complex) is needed primarily to detect slight but potentially dangerous departures from the norm by "self" tissue (cancers), rather than in defence against infection. Those animals most susceptible to this uncontrolled proliferation of cells are likely to be the more complex, active, large and/or long-lived animals and, perhaps, those relying on maximal survival of few offspring. While this makes vertebrates the prime candidate for cancer, by no means all invertebrates are simple, small and short-lived (giant squids, for example)—and invertebrate cancers do exist, although comparatively little is known about them. To date, cases have been most frequently reported in insects and molluscs, but it is uncertain whether these groups are more inclined towards cancer than others, or whether they are simply more frequently studied and/or their tumours more readily identified. More comparative studies on proliferative disorders in diverse phyla should clarify relationships between cancer formation and immunological phenomena. The view might also be taken that the most primitive animals susceptible to cancer mark the phylogenetic level at which specific immune systems emerged, with the proviso that in cases where cancer occurs in age ranges rarely reached under natural conditions, or where mechanisms for "self-cure" exist (autectomy in helminths, for example, where diseased parts are shed and then regenerated), the evolutionary pressure for an immunological "fail-safe" mechanism would be diminished.

The increasing deposition of mesodermal tissue and its derivatives between gut and body surface at the platyhelminth and nemertine levels created a need for circulatory systems in order to maintain efficient nutrition, respiration and excretion. This emergence of circulatory systems in the higher invertebrates must have profoundly affected the defensive network of the body, since pathogens, and possibly cancer cells, could now move with ease to all parts of the animal, thus creating more menace. Hence in the advanced protostomes (especially annelids, molluscs and arthropods) and in advanced deuterostomes (vertebrates) there is a concentrated production of circulating defensive cells, and the formation of strategically located filtering devices to monitor the circulation. Whether such developments of lymphoid/phagocytic organs in the two superphyla are homologous or analogous can only be speculated.

It has been shown that specific tissue incompatibility reactions exist in the coelenterates, though no memory component has so far been demonstrated. In these lowly metazoa there are no blood-vascular or organ systems, and cancers are unlikely to occur: aberrant population breakthroughs would presumably be very rare where there are limited numbers of systems in the body. Similar tissue incompatibility reactions have been described in the phylogenetically distant tunicates. An attractive hypothesis to account for the existence of these tissue incompatibility reactions, at least in crowded stationary colonial forms (e.g. on a coral reef), is that intercolony incompatibility (repulsion) enables genetic and territorial integrity to be maintained, whilst intracolony compatibility (fusion) enhances the structural integrity of the colony. In these circumstances, specificity would be important, but speed of reaction and a memory component less so. It is thus conceivable that, at its most primitive level, the immune system evolved, not to resist infection or cancer, but simply for reasons of space (assuming, of course, that animals with this type of organization were not an evolutionary dead-end).

CHAPTER THREE

AQUATIC VERTEBRATES: AGNATHA

JAWLESS VERTEBRATES (AGNATHA) WERE THE FIRST VERTEBRATES TO APPEAR in the fossil record (figure 3.1). They date from the Ordovician period, about 450 million years ago, and their present-day descendants, the hagfish and lampreys, retain certain features characteristic of this primitive level

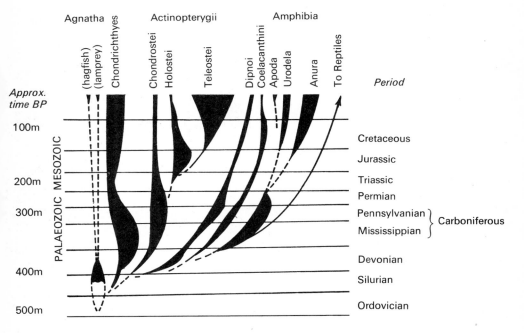

Figure 3.1. Phylogenetic relationships in the fishes and amphibians
The distribution through time of the different groups of fishes and amphibians is shown. BP, time before the present in millions of years. Partly from Romer, A. S. (1966), *Vertebrate Paleontology* (3rd ed.) University of Chicago Press, Chicago (with modifications).

53

of vertebrate evolution. It should, however, be borne in mind that these modern agnathans also show some specialized characteristics: after radiating in the Silurian and Devonian waters for some 100 million years, their armoured ancestors disappeared from the fossil record (presumably superseded by the more efficient jawed fishes which became dominant in the Devonian), leaving only soft-bodied representatives with scavenging and ectoparasitic habits. Since many authors suspect that there has been a long period of separation between the hagfish and lampreys, we shall examine the immunobiology of the two groups individually.

Table 3.1. Comparisons of skin allograft survival times in agnathans and in gnathostome fish*

Animal	Median survival times and ranges First-set (days)	Second-set (days)	Interval between first-set and second-set grafts (days)	Water temperature °C.
AGNATHA				
Hagfish (*Eptatretus stoutii*)	72 (41–140)	28 (18–119)	30	18·5
Lamprey (*Petromyzon marinus*)	38† (21—more than 291)	18† (7—more than 252)	39	18–21
CHONDRICHTHYES				
Stingray (*Dasyatis americana*)	more than 31 (less than 31–53)	less than 12	53	18–28
Horned shark (*Heterodontus francisci*)	41 (27–48)	17 (15–22)	60	22
OSTEICHTHYES				
Paddlefish (*Polyodon spathula*)	42–68 (21—more than 76)	12†	68	18–26 (first-set) 6–13 (second-set)
Arowana (*Osteoglossum bicirrhosum*)	18 (13–25)	5·1 (3–7)	30	25
Goldfish (*Carassius auratus*)	7·2 (6–11)	4·7 (4–6)	25	25
Blue acara (*Aequidens latifrons*)	7·2 (6–11)	4·5 (3–6)	25	25

* From: Hildemann, W. H. (1970), "Transplantation Immunity in Fishes: Agnatha, Chondrichthyes and Osteichthyes," *Transplantation Proceedings*, **11**, 253–259 (with modifications).
† Approximate values.

3.1. Hagfish

Hagfish are marine scavengers, and are unique among the vertebrates in having a high salt concentration in the body fluids, isosmotic with sea water. They are generally regarded as being more primitive than lampreys. Until recently, attempts to demonstrate immune responses in hagfish proved unsuccessful, thus leading to the erroneous belief that they were below the level phylogenetically at which specific immune responses evolved. It has since transpired that the experimental animals were unable to respond, not because of an inherent immunological deficiency, but simply because they were being kept in unsuitable conditions in the laboratory.

3.1.1. Transplantation reactions

It is now established that, provided that they are kept in good uncrowded aquaria and at sufficiently high temperature, hagfish are well able to reject skin allografts. The sequence of observed reactions, including infiltration of the graft bed by lymphocytes, capillary haemorrhage, and whitening of the graft due to pigment cell destruction, is similar to that seen in all other vertebrate groups. Rejection of first-set grafts is invariably prolonged, even at "summer" ocean temperature of 18 °C (see Table 3.1), and lowering of temperature results in even longer graft survival times. However, second-set grafts are rejected more rapidly, indicating immunological memory. The extent and degree of specificity of this memory in hagfish may provide a useful estimation of their immunological "primitiveness".

3.1.2. Antibody production

As in some invertebrate body fluids (see Chapter 2), naturally-occurring heat-labile agglutinins to various vertebrate erythrocytes are regularly found in normal hagfish serum in low titres, and bactericidal substances with low specificity and without a requirement for complement can be rapidly induced. These humoral factors, while providing an interesting link (at least in terms of function) between the vertebrate and invertebrate humoral systems, may not justify the term *antibody* (see Chapters 1 and 2). Nevertheless, other serum factors which are both inducible and specific have been demonstrated, the molecular properties of which are similar to but distinguishable from mammalian IgM. Injection of sheep erythrocytes, for example, elicits specific haemagglutinin titres of up to 1 : 1024 within a three-month period after initial stimulation in animals maintained at 18 °C. Hagfish are thus the first group phylogenetically to show both cell-mediated and antibody responses. Any claims of immunoglobulin homologies with higher vertebrates seem premature, however, particularly in the light of recent lamprey studies (see section 3.2.2). The possibility of secondary antibody responses in hagfish also needs further investigation.

3.1.3. Lymphoid tissues

Circulating lymphocytes have been found in hagfish blood and coelomic fluid and these, along with erythrocytes, may derive from diffuse haemo-poietic foci found in the gut wall. In the genus *Myxine*, other haemo-poietic areas have been described in the anterior kidney, a derivative of the pronephros. This remarkable organ has ciliated ducts (nephrostomes) which drain the coelom and lead into a central mass of fibrous and haemopoietic tissue containing erythrocytes, lymphocytes, granulocytes and phagocytes, and thence into the venous system (see figure 3.2). The central mass is known to trap substances reaching it from the coelom, and would thus be an ideal site for triggering by antigen of immuno-competent cells. In other words, the hagfish pronephros may well function as a true secondary lymphoid organ. However, plasma cells have not been identified here or elsewhere in hagfish, and proliferative responses to antigenic stimulation have so far been seen only in the blood. The

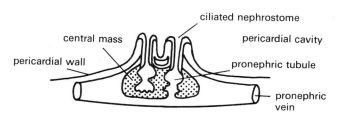

Figure 3.2.   Pronephros of the hagfish *Myxine glutinosa* in the region of the tubules and the central mass

The hagfish pronephros with its tubules and central mass is suspended in the pronephric vein. It acts as a filter in which fluid from the pericardial (coelomic) cavity is led past the central mass into the pronephric vein. The central mass which contains fibrous and haemopoietic tissue is known to trap substances reaching it from the coelom. The diagram (which shows part of the organ) is simplified from the *Myxine* pronephros figured in Holmgren, N. (1950), "On the Pronephros and the Blood in *Myxine glutinosa*", *Acta Zoologica* (Stockholm), **31**, 234–348.

existence and possible location of primary lymphoid tissue (i.e. homo-
logues of the thymus and bursa of Fabricius) also remain matters of
speculation: investigations are hampered by the difficulty in obtaining
developmental stages.

3.2. Lampreys

The adult lamprey is an ectoparasite on fish, but it spends the first few
years of its life history as a mud-burrowing larva, the ammocoete. The
immune system of ammocoetes is of particular interest because their
organization approximates to the generalized vertebrate condition, and
they retain the ancestral habit of filter-feeding.

3.2.1. Transplantation reactions

The capacity of lampreys to reject skin allografts and produce an
accelerated secondary response has been clearly demonstrated (see Table
3.1), both in adults and larvae, though there is a wide variation between
individuals in rejection times. Studies of ammocoete blood lymphocytes
have shown them to be able to undergo blast cell transformation when
cultured *in vitro* at 15 °C with lymphocytes from a second donor (a mixed
lymphocyte reaction), provided that phytohaemagglutinin is present. The
agglutinating properties of phytohaemagglutinin are believed to be
important here (rather than its mitogenic properties) by facilitating surface
contact between lymphocytes. Lampreys, then, clearly have the genetic
capacity to recognize cell-surface (histocompatibility) antigens within the
same species.

3.2.2. Antibody production

Inducible antibodies to several particulate antigens have now been demonstrated in lampreys, subject to maintenance at reasonably high
temperature (e.g. 18 °C); several studies, however, have failed to show
responses induced against soluble antigens. The lamprey antibody is
immunoglobulin, but its relationship to other vertebrate immunoglobulins
is in dispute: some studies have indicated the typical polypeptide structure
of two L (light) chains and two H (heavy) chains (the latter being similar
to the μ-chain of mammalian IgM), others suggest that light chains are
absent. Also, interchain disulphide bonds appear to be lacking. It has
been speculated that the structure of lamprey immunoglobulin might be a

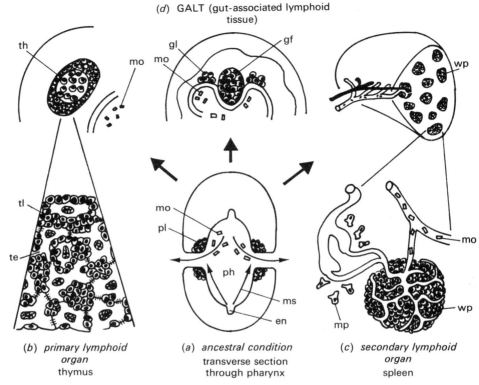

(d) GALT (gut-associated lymphoid tissue)

(b) *primary lymphoid organ* thymus

(a) *ancestral condition* transverse section through pharynx

(c) *secondary lymphoid organ* spleen

Figure 3.3. Phylogeny of vertebrate lymphoid organs

(a) Transverse section through the pharynx of a hypothetical filter-feeding ancestral vertebrate. This is very similar to the condition seen today in the ammocoete larva of the lamprey. Food is filtered from the water current which passes in at the mouth and out through the gill openings, the particles being picked up in a mucus stream (ms) secreted by the endostyle (en). It is possible that pathogenic micro-organisms in this water current (mo, in current indicated by arrows) may also be trapped and held in the pharynx, hence the presence of strategically placed pharyngeal lymphocytic accumulations (pl); lumen of pharynx (ph).

(b) The thymus, which is associated with the pharyngeal epithelium in all jawed vertebrates, consists of a meshwork of branched epithelial cells of pharyngeal origin held together at their desmosomes, with lymphocytes lying in the interstices. As a primary lymphoid organ the thymus is isolated from the main areas of antigen retention: th, thymus showing cortex and medulla; tl, thymic lymphocyte; te, thymic epithelial cell.

(c) The spleen is depicted here as an example of a typical gnathostome secondary lymphoid organ specialized to trap antigen. In the

link between the typical vertebrate immunoglobulin and effector molecules responsible for some of the invertebrate humoral reactions. A more
obvious parallel with invertebrates is the finding in lampreys of a naturally-
occurring haemagglutinin which is not an immunoglobulin. Moreover,
agnathans apparently lack a full complement system capable of effecting
immune haemolysis.

3.2.3. Lymphoid tissues

Haemopoietic tissue is more in evidence in lampreys than in hagfish,
although it is often located in "unusual" areas of the body. We suspect that
such tissue in the ancestral vertebrate became housed in any anatomically
"convenient" spaces. Thus in the present-day lamprey the typhlosole,
which serves primarily to increase the absorptive surface of the gut, also
accommodates blood-forming tissue; this may represent a primitive
spleen. Similarly, haemopoietic cells occupy the soft tissue of the protovertebral arch, an area which lies above, and cushions, the otherwise
poorly protected spinal cord.

As yet we are unsure whether these haemopoietic foci represent stem-
cell-producing tissues, primary or secondary lymphoid organs, or have a
combined function. Although positive identification of stem cells and
primary lymphoid organs is usually difficult experimentally, in a higher
vertebrate a secondary lymphoid organ can readily be shown to trap
injected antigen, and lymphocytes recognizing the antigen are stimulated
to proliferate and form effector cells, such as plasma cells. Although in
lampreys, as in hagfish, plasma cells have not been found, a proliferative
response has been demonstrated, notably in the haemopoietic areas of the
protovertebral arch. This proliferation occurs in clusters, such as one
might expect when clones of cells have been stimulated. On the other
hand, neither the protovertebral arch nor the typhlosole regions show
much uptake of injected antigens, neither does their simple organization

---

spleen, antigen is filtered from the blood (mo, micro-organisms in
the blood stream). The white pulp (wp) is shown in the half spleen
(above) and also in enlarged view (for details see figure 1.13).
Macrophages of the red pulp (mp) line the red pulp sinusoids.
(d) Gut-associated lymphoid tissue (GALT) encounters antigenic
stimulation from the gut lumen (mo, micro-organisms in gut lumen).
It includes compact sub-epithelial follicles (gf) and scattered
lymphocytes lying within the epithelium (gl). While much of this
is secondary lymphoid tissue, a primary lymphoid role for GALT
has also been postulated.

seem particularly suited to the trapping and triggering processes; indeed, the protovertebral arch of at least some ammocoetes is almost devoid of a lymphoid cell population. It is worth noting here that injection of antigen into ammocoetes occasionally induces the appearance *de novo* of simple organs (consisting of blood cells in a connective tissue matrix) which are associated with the vasculature and involved in antigen trapping; however, their appearance could not be correlated with more effective responses.

Other lymphoid accumulations in the lamprey, which have aroused considerable interest, are those associated with the ammocoete pharynx. They consist of placodes lying in the epipharyngeal fold, plus small aggregates of lymphocytes in the submucosa near the external opening of the pharyngeal pouches. The evolution of the lymphoid system may have been influenced by the filter-feeding habit of the ancestral vertebrates: there is a danger to a filter-feeder from pathogenic micro-organisms which may be trapped along with the food particles and held in the pharynx for some time before encountering the digestive enzymes further back in the gut. A functional relationship of this sort, correlated with the need to recognize and deal with foreign organisms invading the pharyngeal epithelium from the trapped food mass, may account for the presence of the lymphoid accumulations in the ammocoete pharynx and for the pharyngeal derivation of the thymus gland in gnathostome (jawed) vertebrates (see figure 3.3). Unfortunately it remains a matter of conjecture whether the ammocoete accumulations really do represent a primitive thymus, since experimental evidence is lacking, and morphological evidence is inconclusive.

3.3. Conclusions

It is now evident that the specific transplantation reaction is a pheno-menon clearly established even in the most primitive members of the vertebrate subphylum and, as work on invertebrates has shown, probably one which has its origins long before the vertebrate stock evolved. On the other hand, present evidence suggests that the ability to synthesize specific antibodies (i.e. immunoglobulins) emerged only with the vertebrates, and even in the Agnatha, homology with the gnathostome immunoglobulin system is rather tenuous. It remains to be seen if immunoglobulin in the form of receptors on the cell surface is responsible for specific recognition by Agnatha, as is believed to be the case in higher vertebrates.

While hagfish and lampreys appear to possess the basic functional requirements of the vertebrate immune system (e.g. specificity, memory, proliferation), there is a lack of structural sophistication and differentiation of their lymphoid system which may reflect limitations in the spectrum and vigour of their responses. It is still problematical whether there is any real separation at this phylogenetic level between stem-cell-producing tissues, primary and secondary lymphoid organs. However, the ammocoete pharynx may show the beginnings of an intimate association between epithelial and lymphoid cells, an association which plays a crucial role in the thymus of gnathostomes.

CHAPTER FOUR

AQUATIC VERTEBRATES: CARTILAGINOUS AND BONY FISHES

AS THE EARLIEST JAWED VERTEBRATES, FISHES RADIATED IN THE PALAEOZOIC and by the Devonian period had already given rise to three main lines, one of cartilaginous fish (Chondrichthyes) and two lines of bony fish (Osteichthyes). Of the two lines of bony fish, the Actinopterygii form the majority of present-day bony fishes, the Sarcopterygii have only a few modern representatives, e.g. Dipnoi, Coelacanthini, but are the group which gave rise to the tetrapods (see figure 3.1.).

4.1. Chondrichthyes

Although present-day elasmobranchs (sharks and rays) look very different from their heavily-armoured ancestors, and attempts to interpret their immunological status in terms of early fish evolution must needs be tentative, they and the lower orders of bony fishes may at least provide some clues about the basic immunological characteristics of the early gnathostomes.

4.1.1. *Transplantation reactions*

As in Agnatha, rejection of first-set skin allografts by cartilaginous fish is long-term (chronic) in nature, even at elevated water temperatures (see Table 3.1). Repeated grafting can, however, lead to progressively more rapid rejection.

4.1.2. *"In vitro" responses*

A failure by nurse sharks (*Ginglymostoma*) and horned sharks (*Hetero-dontus*) to produce a mixed lymphocyte reaction has been reported, but it remains to be seen whether the failure to respond has a phylogenetic or technical basis. Lymphocytes from nurse sharks proliferate when mixed with bovine gamma globulin (BGG) antigen in culture, provided that they come from a shark which has been previously immunized with BGG. This reponse is specific, since it is inhibited by shark anti-BGG serum. Lymphocytes taken from peripheral blood of nurse sharks respond *in vitro* to the non-specific mitogen concanavalin A. In addition, cells which form the bottom layer when blood lymphocytes are separated experimentally in a Ficoll-Isopaque gradient, can be stimulated by phytohaemagglutinin (PHA). Reactivity to this latter non-specific mitogen (PHA), however, is inhibited by other lymphocytes which are present in normal blood. The interest of these observations is that they indicate that a heterogeneity amongst lymphocytic populations, which is readily apparent in higher vertebrates, is already present in the fishes.

4.1.3. *Antibody production*

This is a well-studied area of shark immunology: their large size makes it possible (but dangerous?) to obtain good quantities of serum for analysis.

Immunoglobulin classes

The typical basic 2H-2L chain structure characteristic of mammalian immunoglobulins is already present at the elasmobranch level. Furthermore, a pentapeptide sequence has been conserved in the variable region of L chains of immunoglobulin from animals as widely separated as sharks, birds and mammals, with a similar but less highly conserved sequence in the variable region of H chains. Such conservation is remarkable in view of the period of time (about 400 million years) since sharks and mammals diverged.

In several species of shark, immunoglobulin has been shown to occur in two molecular sizes, 17–19S (pentameric form) and 7S (monomeric). These are known to possess one antigen-binding site per 2H-2L unit, but there may be an additional binding site present which has escaped detection due to low affinity (poor fit) for antigen. The 19S and 7S immunoglobulins are believed by most workers to represent only a single immunoglobulin class (IgM) because their H chains are considered to be of the same type (μ-chains). However, a recent report claims to have found antigenic (therefore structural) differences in immunoglobulin H chains within a number of species of galeoid sharks and one squaloid species, hence more than one class of shark immunoglobulin. These recent findings, if substantiated, suggest that different immunoglobulin classes in higher animals could have arisen from different immediate molecular ancestors rather than from a single "most primitive" immunoglobulin, hitherto presumed to be IgM.

Molecules homologous to the J chain (see section 1.4.2) have been observed in IgM polymers of both elasmobranch and actinopterygian fish; indeed, these joining chains appear to regulate the degree of polymerization of the immunoglobulins of all jawed vertebrates.

Ontogeny of elasmobranch immunoglobulins

Immunoglobulin constitutes about 50% of the serum protein of an adult nurse shark, but only about 1% in the newborn; in these, other proteins compensate to maintain osmotic pressure. The few immunoglobulins present at birth are 19S, with 7S immunoglobulin appearing only later, and both types slowly but progressively increase in concentration. Since there is no evidence that the 7S immunoglobulin is either a precursor or a degradation product of the 19S, and there are no foetal-maternal connections, the two immunoglobulins must both be of foetal origin and synthesized independently of each other. As in mammals, the high-molecular-weight (19S) immunoglobulin is largely restricted to an intravascular role, whereas 7S equilibrates throughout the plasma volume.

Induced and natural antibodies

The most readily detectable inducible antibodies in elasmobranchs are of the 19S type: primary immunization of nurse sharks with *Salmonella* elicits 19S (high-molecular-weight) antibody after 30 days, whereas 7S (low-molecular-weight) antibodies were isolated only after nearly a year of immunization at 25 °C. Results of this sort caution against bald assumptions regarding the immunological armoury of poikilothermic species purely on the basis of short-term findings. The ability of sharks to respond more vigorously following a secondary antigenic stimulation has also been demonstrated, although this occurs only to some antigens and may in part be a doze effect. It seems doubtful that all the quantitative and qualitative parameters of the mammalian secondary antibody response are present in elasmobranchs.

In addition to experimentally induced antibodies, naturally-occurring factors have been found in shark serum which can react with a great variety of antigens. Their effects include neutralization of viruses, killing of bacteria, and lysis and agglutination of erythrocytes of many species.

This natural reactivity of sharks, unlike that in invertebrates, resembles classical antibody at least insofar as most of it is associated with macroglobulin (19S) and the lytic reactions involve complement. It is possible that sharks are reacting to an antigenic determinant which is shared by a large variety of antigens in the environment, and that the polyspecific reactivity of their serum is merely a reflection of such a recognition.

4.1.4. *Lymphoid tissues*

Cartilaginous fishes—and indeed all vertebrates except Agnatha—show clear morphological evidence of a thymus. In some embryonic elasmobranchs (e.g. rays), all six pharyngeal pouches including the spiracular pouch, can give rise to thymic buds from the dorsal epithelium (near the junction of the outpushing endodermal pouch and the ingrowing ectodermal groove), although these buds do not all contribute to the adult thymus (see figure 4.1). The thymus, although epithelial in origin, becomes lymphoid early in ontogeny and differentiates a cortex (consisting of densely populated small lymphocytes) and medulla; it also separates from the pharyngeal epithelium to lie free in the mesenchyme.

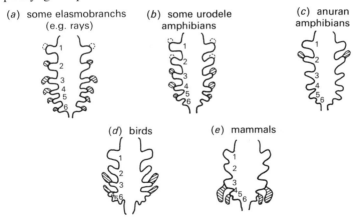

Figure 4.1.   **Diagrams of the pharynx showing the origin of the thymus in different vertebrate groups**
The paired pharyngeal pouches are numbered 1–6. The thymus is shown as a bud; this is hatched in the diagram where the thymic bud contributes to the formation of the definitive thymus, and dotted for rudiments which disappear without yielding adult derivatives. Partly from Brachet, A. (1921), *Traité d'Embryologie des Vertébrés*, Masson et Cie, Paris, and from Romer, A. S. (1970), *The Vertebrate Body*, 4th ed., W. B. Saunders Company, Philadelphia and London. Mainly after Maurer.

Apart from a definitive thymus, cartilaginous fish also possess a discrete spleen. This is encapsulated and differentiated into a red pulp with blood sinuses and a lymphocytic white pulp. Haemopoietic areas are also found in the gut wall and kidneys, and more restrictedly in gonads, cranial region and heart wall. In general these haemopoietic tissues have a mixed character, i.e. they generate several kinds of blood cells (lymphocytes, granulocytes, erythrocytes). Little attention has been paid to the nature and tissue location of antibody-forming cells in elasmobranchs, although experiments showing good antibody responses to both intravenously and subcutaneously injected antigen in splenectomized sharks have demonstrated that the most obvious site, the spleen, cannot be the only or major one involved in antibody production. Cells with the morphological characteristics of plasma cells have been found in advanced elasmobranchs (e.g. leopard shark and nurse shark) but not in primitive representatives such as the horned shark and guitarfish; but whether this has any functional significance remains to be determined.

4.2. Osteichthyes

The immunology of the Actinopterygii (ray-finned fishes), particularly the teleosts, has been fairly well investigated, a reflection no doubt of their availability and economic importance. They are, however, an independent line of evolution. The Sarcopterygii (lobe-finned fishes, including the Crossopterygii and the Dipnoi) are closer to the tetrapod line, but unfortunately our knowledge of the immune systems of this group is still fragmentary. The present section therefore deals mainly with the immunobiology of the ray-finned bony fishes.

4.2.1. *Transplantation reactions*

Most teleosts are capable of a rapid (acute) rejection of first-set skin allografts, and repeated grafting leads to good development and persistence of specific memory (see Table 3.1). These responses are as vigorous as those of many higher vertebrates; similar histological events accompany the reaction (lymphocytic infiltration, capillary haemorrhage and pigment-cell destruction) and there is impressive polymorphism of the histocompatibility genes. Graft rejection times are slower (sub-acute) in a less advanced teleost, the arowana, *Osteoglossum bicirrhosum*, and slower still in the paddlefish, *Polyodon spathula*, a member of the Chondrostei, the most primitive group of actinopterygian fishes. In fact, graft rejection in the paddlefish is more akin to that seen in Agnatha and Chondrichthyes (see Table 3.1).

Temperature effects

As in other poikilothermic vertebrates, the onset of an allograft rejection in fish, and the speed with which they destroy the graft, are temperature-dependent. At low temperatures the rejection of the first-set grafts is inhibited to a greater degree than rejection of second-set grafts.

Ontogeny of transplantation reactivity

Larval teleosts, like larval lampreys, are able to respond to histo-compatibility antigens. Allogeneic fin grafts placed on a 2-day old sword-tail (*Xiphophorus*), for example, are rejected within 11 days. Similarly in the viviparous surf perch (*Cymatogaster*), allograft incompatibility is expressed soon after birth.

Ontogenetic appearance of histocompatibility antigens

Histocompatibility antigens are present even in embryonic fish: prior implantation of a teleost embryo into the body cavity of an unrelated adult fish causes the accelerated rejection by that fish of scale grafts taken from the embryo's mother; while prior transplantation of adult tissues leads to an accelerated rejection of implanted related embryos. This can create problems for species of viviparous fish—and for any viviparous vertebrate—since during gestation the foetus is in a position, relative to the mother, analogous to that of an allograft of tissue. In the Poeciliidae (a family which includes live-bearers such as the guppy), the site of gestation, the ovary, lacks any special properties which would make it a favourable site for allograft survival; protection of the foetus is afforded by the fertilization membrane. At the end of pregnancy, rupture of the membrane, release of the embryo from the ovarian follicle, and its passage to the exterior, all occur rapidly, before a maternal alloimmune reaction can be effected. A similar potential problem exists where sperms are stored in the ovary of viviparous fish to allow the production of several broods from a single insemination. In this case, however, the complete explanation for survival of the allograft is not at hand.

4.2.2. *"In vitro" responses*

Teleost lymphocytes show proliferative responses when cultured *in vitro* with specific antigen. Thus lymphocytes taken from gray snappers, *Lutjanus griseus* which have been immunized with a viral antigen, respond to this antigen *in vitro* by an increased incorporation of thymidine. Teleost lymphocytes also show proliferative responses to the non-specific mitogens concanavalin A, phytohaemagglutinin (PHA) and lipopolysaccharide (LPS). Evidence for mixed lymphocyte reactivity is conflicting: a repeated failure to respond has been reported for gray snappers, while significant responses have been demonstrated in trout.

4.2.3. *Humoral immunity in Actinopterygii*

Immunoglobulin classes

The predominant immunoglobulin in Actinopterygii is a high-molecular-weight form (approximately 14S) which, unlike other vertebrate macroglobulins, is tetrameric rather than pentameric. Studies on the tetrameric antibody of the giant grouper (*Epinephelus*) have suggested a valence of 8, with 4 high- and 4 low-affinity antigen-binding sites per molecule, though in carp (*Cyprinus*) a total of only 4 combining sites per tetramer has so far been detected. Grouper and carp tetramers have been identified as IgM. However, goldfish (*Carassius*) immunized with bovine serum albumin (BSA) can produce two immunoglobulins of similar size (16·4S and 15·3S) but antigenically distinguishable, and perch (*Perca*) immunized with human gamma globulin (HGG) or chicken erythrocytes produce two immunoglobulins both of 14·5S but differing in sensitivity to 2-mercaptoethanol. There is thus some evidence of structural heterogeneity in teleost macroglobulins.

In some but not all of the teleosts so far studied, low-molecular-weight (approximately 7S) immunoglobulins have been identified, as well as tetrameric forms. Monomeric antibody has also been found in the bowfin (*Amia*), a member of the Holostei (a group intermediate between Chondrostei and Teleostei), although in the gar (*Lepisosteus*), a member of the same group, only tetrameric immunoglobulin has been detected. In experiments where low-molecular-weight antibodies have been found, their appearance during the course of immunization may or may not supersede that of polymeric antibody. In the goldfish, for example, antibacteriophage activity was evenly distributed between high and low-molecular-weight antibodies at two months after stimulation, but at 5 months they were almost entirely of low molecular weight. This polymer-monomer sequence is similar to that seen in sharks and higher vertebrates. On the other hand, in groupers producing antibodies to dinitrophenol (DNP), both high and low-molecular-weight immunoglobulin types were found at various intervals between one month and two years after immunization. It seems likely that at least some of these monomeric immunoglobulins are precursors or breakdown products of larger molecules; others may prove to be quite separate entities.

One aspect of immunoglobulin structure which has been compared phylogenetically only in the trout is the depth of the antigen-binding site. It has recently been found that the depth of the hapten-combining site of trout anti-DNP antibody is similar to that in the rabbit (11·5 Å).

Secondary antibody responses

The ability to produce an enhanced antibody response following a repeated antigenic stimulation has been reported for the holostean *Lepisosteus* (immunized with diphtheria toxoid or alum-precipitated bovine serum albumin (BSA)) and for the teleost *Haemulon*, the margate (immunized with BSA) but in both cases antibody was associated throughout with macroglobulin; unlike the higher vertebrates, no qualitative effects involving a shift in synthesis from one antibody type to another were observed. In the goldfish, however, a qualitative effect of secondary immunization (with BSA) has been claimed, in addition to accelerated responses and higher titres: two distinct macroglobulin antibodies were produced sequentially after the primary injection, but simultaneously after a repeated injection.

Complement

As in elasmobranchs, there is evidence of a conventional antibody-complement system in bony fish, although complement from the same or a closely related species seems to be required. Studies on salmonid sera suggest that fish complement components may be more uniform in molecular size than in mammals and that the system as a whole is less complex.

Secretory antibodies

There is good evidence in Actinopterygii that antibodies from their secretions are very similar, perhaps identical, to those in the serum. Antibodies present in plaice (*Pleuronectes*) serum and mucus, for example, are both of high molecular weight and have similar carbohydrate and amino-acid compositions; in chub (*Leuciscus*), anti-acanthocephalan precipitins in the serum and in epidermal and gut mucus are all of high molecular weight (17S), are all sensitive to 2-mercaptoethanol and show antigenic identity; and antibody in mucus of the gar (*Lepisosteus*) has several properties (e.g. molecular weight, sensitivity to 2-mercaptoethanol) in common with the serum macroglobulin. It seems clear, therefore, that fish lack a separate class of secretory antibody at all comparable with the IgA of mammals.

Studies on plaice have shown that the presence of antibody in the secretions may result from local synthesis or from transudation from the serum, depending on the route of entry by antigen. Administration of heat-killed *Vibrio* bacteria parenterally (via the intraperitoneal or subcutaneous route) elicited high antibody titres in the serum and low titres also in the cutaneous and gut mucus, suggesting that the secretory antibody derived from the serum. On the other hand, after oral administration of *Vibrio* by mixing it with the food, antibody appeared in gut mucus in significantly higher titres than in serum, suggesting that in this case its synthesis occurred in close proximity to the mucous surface. This ability to immunize fish orally by mixing antigen with their food offers important commercial possibilities in fish farming, where large numbers of fish need to be maintained in healthy condition. However, oral immunization may not necessarily prove effective for those pathogens which normally enter the body by another route. Moreover, as the hagfish story (section 3.1) has demonstrated, the immunological capability of fish can also be enhanced simply by improving their environmental conditions.

Temperature effects

Antibody responses in fish are generally suppressed by low temperatures, but reactivity can be detected in cold-water species. Thus the sablefish *Anaplopoma fimbria* from the cold waters of the North Pacific produces antibodies at 5–8 °C, whereas the warm-water carp *Cyprinus carpio* produces antibodies at 20–25 °C, but none if maintained throughout at 12 °C. Interestingly, carp which are immunized at 25 °C and then transferred to 12 °C can synthesize and release antibody at this low temperature. It has been suggested that this phenomenon may have some natural value in the resistance of fish to pathogens commonly encountered in their environment, since their immune response might otherwise be depressed in the cold season.

Other experiments in which carp have been moved from one temperature to another during the time course of a response suggest that the initial steps of phagocytosis, metabolic processing and recognition of the antigen are independent of ambient temperature. Thus fish stimulated with antigen in the cold and then moved to a higher temperature can produce antibody after only a short latent period, suggesting that some of the earlier events in the response must have occurred at the lower temperature. The temperature-dependent stages appear to be those involving the cellular interactions and differentiation processes which lead to antibody production.

Natural humoral factors

It might be argued that a low temperature which restricts antibody production in a poikilotherm would also decrease the activity of pathogens. Nevertheless fish can be overcome by various diseases in a shorter time than that required for them to produce a measurable immune response. In such situations "natural" factors, found in normal healthy fish, may play a significant role. These factors include a heterogeneous collection of agglutinins, lysins and precipitins. Specificity is variable: a non-antibody factor called C-reactive protein found recently in plaice will precipitate with extracts prepared from bacteria, fungi and nematodes, while natural haemagglutinins obtained, for example, from the fresh-water catfish *Tandanus* are specific towards antigens of the human ABO blood group system. The latter, like natural haemagglutinins in sharks, appear to be macroglobulins. Similarly the long-nose gar, *Lepisosteus osseus*, possesses high-molecular-weight natural agglutinins, together with natural haemolysins which participate with complement. Several of these natural factors thus share some of the characteristics of typical induced antibodies. It is also true, however, that some vertebrate proteins with specific receptor sites for certain polysaccharides or foreign erythrocytes (eel anti-O and lamprey haemagglutinins, for example) are structurally quite distinct from the known immunoglobulins.

Immediate hypersensitivity reactions

Immediate hypersensitivity reactions are mediated by antibodies capable of attaching to target cells such as mast cells (see figure 1.5) and releasing pharmacologically active agents. In certain species of marine flatfish, including the plaice *Pleuronectes platessa*, some fungal extracts cause an immediate erythema (reddening of the skin) when injected intra-dermally. This reaction can be passively transferred to a non-reactive species, the flounder, *Platichthyes flesus*, by injecting serum from the plaice. The results suggest that an immediate hypersensitivity reaction is occurring in these flatfish. It is not yet known which serum components are responsible. There may be an as yet unidentified tissue-fixing antibody, or possibly a non-immunoglobulin factor, C-reactive protein, is involved.

4.2.4. *Immunoglobulin classes of Dipnoi*

Lungfish, which are distant relations of the tetrapods (see figure 3.1), have a similar pentameric form of IgM, plus a monomeric immunoglobulin of a different class. Both the African lungfish *Protopterus aethiopus* and the Australian lungfish *Neoceratodus forsteri* possess this latter low-molecular-weight type of immunoglobulin which has been tentatively designated IgN. IgN sediments at 5·8–5·9S. Its heavy chain differs from the heavy chain (μ-chain) of IgM in both its physical and antigenic properties; its molecular weight is 38,000, compared with 70,000 for the μ-chain of IgM. At this level of evolution, therefore, we begin to see a distinct heterogeneity of the immunoglobulin classes.

4.2.5. *Lymphoid tissues*

Morphology

All bony fish possess a thymus. This organ displays a remarkably similar histological picture throughout the jawed vertebrates, and bony fish are no exception in their possession of typical paired thymic organs with cortical and medullary organization. Hassall's corpuscles are present in the thymus of fishes as in that of higher vertebrates. These are concentrically organized multicellular or unicellular structures; in mammals they have been shown to localize antigen.

The "living fossil" crossopterygian *Latimeria* (coelacanth) shows a well-developed lobulated thymus which, as in Dipnoi, does not apparently involute, while the sturgeon *Acipenser*, a primitive actinopterygian, again shows a distinct lobed thymus, but one which degenerates with age. The latter condition is perhaps more typical of vertebrates in general. The teleost thymus, though it does involute at sexual maturity, is peculiar in that it does not detach from the pharyngeal epithelium from which it derived. Thymic development in Dipnoi on the other hand is very similar to that in amphibians.

With the exception of the thymus, haemopoietic tissues of bony fish, like those of elasmobranchs, are non-specialized—and are strictly speaking more than just lymphoid—since they are also involved in the production of blood cells other than lymphocytes. There is, nevertheless, some degree of sophistication, notably in the spleen: this is differentiated

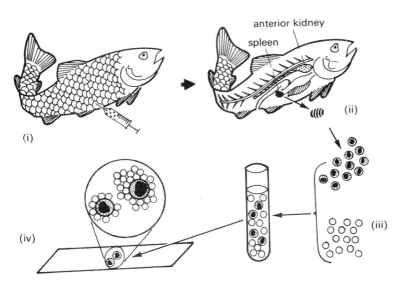

Figure 4.2. Immunocytoadherence (rosette formation)
Immunocytoadherence detects antibody on single cells. It can be applied in experiments where foreign erythrocytes or bacteria are used as antigens. Cells with surface receptors for determinants on the antigenic cells will bind the cells to form a single-layered rosette. Those which are secreting antibody will also bind antigenic cells further from the central rosette and so form a multi-layered cluster.

In the experiment shown here, a fish is immunized with sheep erythrocytes (i), lymphoid tissue (e.g. the spleen) is removed (ii), its cells suspended and mixed with the erythrocytes (iii), and after a suitable incubation period (e.g. overnight at 4 °C) placed on a counting slide and examined microscopically (iv). The enlarged view (circled) shows a lymphoid cell surrounded by a single layer of sheep erythrocytes (a single-layered rosette) on the left and a lymphoid cell with a cluster of sheep erythrocytes (a multi-layered rosette) on the right. These lymphoid cells are termed rosette-forming cells (RFCs).

into red pulp and white pulp and, except in the Dipnoi, lies outside the confines of the gut as a discrete organ. Distinct gut-associated foci are also found in most fish, and it is suspected (but not proven) that these may be involved in local antibody synthesis, e.g. that secreted with the gut mucus. Other haemopoietic tissue is found extensively in teleost pronephroi, and to a lesser degree on the surface of dipnoan kidneys, although it is lacking in the *Latimeria* kidney. Foci have also been reported associated with the heart and gonads of diverse species.

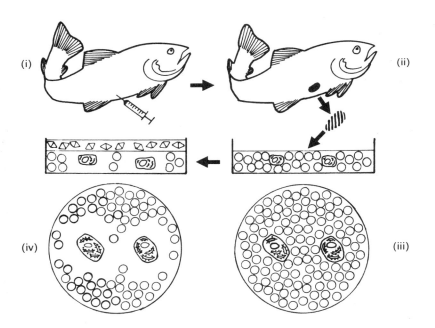

Figure 4.3.   Local haemolysis in agar gel (Jerne-Nordin technique)
Individual antibody-forming cells can be identified using this method of plaque formation. An animal is immunized with foreign erythrocytes (i), lymphoid tissue is removed (ii), its cells suspended and plated on soft agar to which the erythrocytes used for immunization have been added (iii) (depicted in the diagram in side view and from above). On incubation, the antibody-forming cells release their immunoglobulin which coats the surrounding antigenic cells. Complement is then added (indicated by double triangles) and lysis of the coated erythrocytes occurs, leaving a clear area (plaque) around each antibody-forming cell (iv). The antibody-forming cells are termed plaque-forming cells (PFCs).

Antibody synthesis

Plasma cells identified purely on morphological criteria have been identified in all groups of Actinopterygii. However, techniques which permit identification of cells forming antibody to bacterial or erythrocytic antigens by means of immunocytoadherence (figure 4.2) or plaque formation (figure 4.3) question the significance of fish plasma cells in antibody production. For example, in perch immunized with *Salmonella adelaide* flagella, over 80% of the antibody-forming cells from the spleen between 3 and 7 days after injection were small to medium lymphocytes, and the rest were large blast cells; plasma cells were only occasionally seen. Cell proliferation occurred in the population of larger cells. In trout spleen and pronephros, cells responding to sheep erythrocytes include small and larger lymphocytes as well as plasma cells.

In teleosts the spleen and pronephros are the major sites of antibody synthesis, as shown by the number of antibody-forming cells they contain, although in these fish, as in elasmobranchs, the spleen is not essential for antibody production: splenectomy of gray snappers *Lutjanus griseus* does not appear to affect their ability to elicit circulating antibodies to subcutaneously or intravenously injected antigen (bovine serum albumin). As in hagfish (*Myxine*), the association of lymphoid tissue with the kidney in teleosts may result from the filtration of antigen: the cord-like arrangement of lymphoid tissue in the bluegill (*Lepomis*) pronephros is remarkably similar to that in the mammalian lymph node. Notwithstanding this analogy, no tissue exists in fish which corresponds in location or derivation to mammalian lymph nodes.

Surface immunoglobulins

This area of study in fish and other poikilotherms is in its infancy. Fluorescent studies (see figure 4.4), employing rabbit anti-carp IgM antiserum have, however, demonstrated immunoglobulin on the surface of carp lymphocytes. In the blood and the pronephros, 30–58% of the lymphocytes showed immunoglobulin "caps" on their surface, while in the spleen 25–45% of the lymphocytes displayed these surface-associated immunoglobulins, and in the thymus the proportion was over 65%. The presence of a mixed population of lymphocytes in the carp thymus (i.e. immunoglobulin-bearing and non-immunoglobulin-bearing) contrasts with the mouse thymus where the proportion of immunoglobulin-bearing lymphocytes is negligible, but the significance of this is as yet obscure. The "caps"

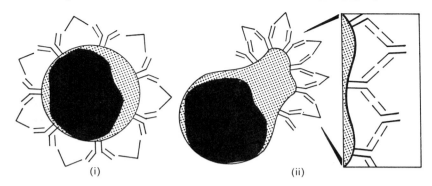

Figure 4.4. Immunoglobulin on the surface of lymphocytes demonstrated by immunofluorescence

When a lymphocyte reacts with a fluorescent labelled antiserum raised against the immunoglobulin of the species, the surface of the lymphocyte is stained, initially with diffuse fluorescence. In diagram (i), divalent antibody (represented as broad Vs) is depicted in combination with the surface immunoglobulin of the cell (represented as 2H-2L molecules). This stage is followed quite rapidly by the aggregation of the fluorescence into patches which coalesce to form a "cap" at one pole of the lymphocyte, probably being swept together in the moving membrane of the cell (ii). The enlarged view of the polar "cap" (in rectangle) shows the 2H-2L immunoglobulin of the fluorescent antiserum in more detail, cross-linking the membrane-associated immunoglobulin molecules of the lymphocyte. With further incubation the complex is taken into the cytoplasm, and the surface staining disappears. Its reappearance after incubation in fresh medium indicates that surface immunoglobulin is actively synthesized by the lymphocyte and not merely adsorbed.

can be re-formed *in vitro*, a finding which indicates that the surface immunoglobulin is actively synthesized by the cell and not merely adsorbed.

The fate of circulating lymphocytes

Classic studies on lymphocyte traffic in rodents have been achieved by removing lymphocytes from a lymphatic duct, labelling them radioactively *in vitro*, then injecting them into syngeneic individuals to study their migration pathways. In the lower vertebrates as a rule, inbred strains are not available, and to prevent destruction of donor lymphocytes, the latter must be injected into the same individuals from which they came. Such a procedure has recently been achieved in plaice. Results have shown many points of similarity with lymphocyte migrations in rodents: in particular, no significant numbers of labelled cells penetrated the thymus; the majority lodged in the secondary lymphoid organs (spleen and kidney). Unlike rodents, however, a recirculation of lymphoid cells between blood and lymph via the secondary lymphoid organs could not be demonstrated in the plaice.

4.3. Conclusions

Teleosts, as masters of the aquatic environment, are as diverse and highly specialized in their own right as the higher tetrapods are on land. The findings that their immune systems are both efficient (e.g. the rapidity of graft rejection) and peculiar (e.g. the tetrameric nature of their immuno-globulin) are thus not unexpected. Nevertheless, we can see that certain features, notably the possession of a definitive thymus and the typical 2H-2L immunoglobulin chain structure, are fundamental attributes of the gnathostome immune system, since they have been conserved in the bony and cartilaginous fishes as a whole.

While the tissue transplant immunity of teleosts appears to be as highly developed as in mammals (provided the former are maintained at sufficiently high temperature), graft rejection in less highly evolved Actino-pterygii and in Chondrichthyes and Agnatha is much slower even at optimal temperature. There is thus evidence of a phylogenetic progression from chronic through to acute rejection.

Despite the remarkable similarities between fish and mammalian anti-bodies in terms of their basic chain structure and the frequency of antigen-binding sites per molecule, to date only one of the mammalian-type immunoglobulin classes (IgM) has been positively and uniformly identified in fish. In view of this, and of the demonstration of μ-chains in agnathans, IgM is considered as the "original" immunoglobulin class. Nonetheless, recent claims of immunoglobulin heterogeneity in elasmobranchs and some of the advanced bony fish surely warrant further investigation. More detailed studies on fish complement and "natural antibody" molecules are also needed.

The functional organization of the lymphoid tissues in fish is a further area which awaits more detailed investigation, although in teleosts at least there is good evidence that the spleen and pronephros are important sites of antibody synthesis, and that plasma cells are by no means the only cell type involved. Apart from the morphological evidence of a thymus, we know very little of a possible stem cell-primary-secondary lymphoid hierarchy in fish (see section 1.7.1) or of an associated heterogeneity of lymphocyte function, although evidence for some functional heterogeneity amongst lymphocytic populations in fish is now emerging. At the moment we can only speculate that the appearance of a thymus in the ancestral gnathostomes (which probably possessed one dorsal thymus per pharyngeal pouch) heralded the specialized roles in which homoiotherm T-cells are implicated.

CHAPTER FIVE

EMERGENCE ON TO LAND:
THE AMPHIBIANS—URODELA AND APODA

AMPHIBIANS EVOLVED FROM FRESH-WATER ANCESTORS CAPABLE OF breathing air. Many adapt well to the conditions of laboratory aquaria and vivaria and, in consequence, they have been widely used for a variety of physiological and developmental studies. They also possess a number of features which make them especially suitable for immunological investigations. In particular, techniques devised for experimental embryology of amphibians have been put to good use in studies on the ontogeny of the immune system. The early developmental stages are readily accessible and easy to manipulate, good cell markers can be produced by the creation of polyploid forms, and convenient culture methods are available for the study of immune responses *in vitro*. Even the very young larval stages can readily withstand surgical operations, e.g. that of early removal of the thymus. In addition, many amphibians can be kept in healthy condition in the laboratory during long-term experiments, such as those involving immunization schedules and immunological memory; they can also be held at varying body temperatures.

Amphibians are not unique in the possession of some of these practical advantages but their general acceptance as laboratory animals has resulted in their being the best studied group of poikilotherms, especially in certain aspects of their immunobiology, such as transplantation immunity, the ontogeny of immunocompetence, and the role of the lymphoid organs.

We shall deal with amphibian immunobiology at some length since, besides the wealth of information accumulated as a consequence of the group's technical suitability, genuine immunological innovations have arisen at this turning point in vertebrate evolution.

The amphibians emerged on to land some 350 million years ago. They flourished in the late Palaeozoic era, but are represented today by only three Orders (or perhaps four Orders if the sirens are removed from the Order Urodela and placed into a separate Order, Trachystomata).

Amphibians of the Orders Urodela and Apoda (=Caecilia) are in several respects more primitive than those of the Order Anura, and this is reflected in their immunobiology. The anurans undergo a more radical process of metamorphosis than that seen in other amphibians, and their immune system is considerably more advanced. They are therefore discussed separately in the next chapter (Chapter 6).

5.1. Urodela and apoda

The apodans are an aberrant group of legless amphibians adapted for burrowing. They retain, in reduced form, the scales of their early ancestors. Apart from some work on graft rejection, their immunobiology has been little investigated. In contrast, extensive reports are available for urodeles, particularly in the field of transplantation immunity, where a number of species from four families (mud puppies, newts, tiger salamanders and axolotls, and the lungless dusky salamanders) have been studied.

5.1.1. *Transplantation reactions*

First-set responses

Rejection of skin grafts in urodeles follows a sequence of events similar to that of other vertebrates. It is usually a prolonged process in this group. Typically, an allograft at first heals in well and is fully viable. After some one to three weeks, blood vessels in the graft area dilate, and lymphocytes accumulate in the graft region. Rejection takes about another three weeks, during which time the degree of lymphocytic infiltration of the graft is roughly proportional to the amount of graft cell death.

Destruction of the pigment cells (melanophores) is readily observed, and this gives a useful indication of the end point of graft rejection. In many urodeles the process takes 30–55 days (at 20–25 °C) but individual survival times range widely (from 7 to 400 days) and some grafts appear to be tolerated indefinitely. A histocompatibility reaction of this sort, where grafts show a median survival time (MST) of about a month or more, is termed *chronic rejection*. This is in contrast to *acute rejection* (which occurs within about two weeks) or *subacute rejection* (in about the third week after application of the graft).

Alloimmune responses in urodeles are probably effected solely by weak histocompatibility reactions. Both the strength and the number of disparate histocompatibility antigens are important in determining the rate of graft rejection, and the prolonged survival times in this group are believed to be due to lack of a major histocompatibility locus, possibly together with a high degree of antigen sharing, and enhancement. Xenografts, as well as allografts, usually show chronic rejection patterns.

Chronic rejection also occurs in the Apoda. In experiments on *Typhlonectes compressicaudata* (which unlike most apodans is a fully aquatic form), the recorded survival times of first-set allografts ranged from 10 to 161 days with an MST of 29 days at 25 °C. Thus urodeles and apodans resemble the agnathans, chondrichthian fish and primitive bony fish in their prolonged process of graft rejection. These groups (and the reptiles—see Chapter 7) apparently lack a major (strong) histocompatibility complex similar to that of the H-2 system of the mouse.

Second-set responses

Immunological memory in urodeles has been clearly demonstrated by the accelerated rejection of second-set allografts. Experiments on the alpine newt *Triturus alpestris* revealed a vigorous and typical memory response in which first-set skin grafts were rejected with an MST of 27 days, whereas second-set grafts from the same donor were rejected in 8 days (MST). Similarly the Japanese newt *Cynops pyrrhogaster* showed an accelerated second-set response to skin allografts, the MST for first-set grafts being 42·6 days and that for second-set grafts 19·4 days (at 20 °C). Studies on the red-spotted or common American newt *Notophthalmus viridescens* (also, now incorrectly, classified as *Diemictylus viridescens* or *Triturus viridescens*) indicate that alloimmune transplantation memory is long-lived. Accelerated rejection was still shown when the second-set graft was applied three months after rejection of the first-set graft (at 25 °C).

It has also been demonstrated in this species that multiple transplantations from the same donor can progressively immunize a recipient, so that an eventual minimal survival time is shown not by the second-set but by the third-set, or occasionally even the fourth-set graft. This differs from acute rejection patterns (where the MST reached by the second-set exposure usually shows no further reduction) but it has been reported for chronic rejection in other vertebrate classes and it also typifies the transplantation memory of some invertebrates.

Repeat grafts on urodeles sometimes show instances of prolonged, rather than curtailed, survival. This phenomenon (which has been described in the apodan *Typhlonectes compressicaudata* as well as in urodeles) may reflect true negative memory (tolerance) or there may be active enhancement of graft survival mediated by enhancing antibodies.

An alternative unusual method for eliminating foreign tissue has been described for the newt *Notophthalmus viridescens*. In this response allogeneic tissue transplanted subcutaneously is extruded through ruptures in the epidermis. The reaction has an immunological basis; this is indicated by the retention of autoimplants and the greater incidence of extrusion in second-set reactions than for first-set implants. It may well have evolved in relation to the elimination of parasites, and perhaps derives from the more primitive encapsulation mechanisms of the invertebrates by addition of an immune-mediated extrusion process.

5.1.2. Tolerance induction

The ease with which tolerance can be induced in urodeles is a phenomenon known for many years and extensively utilized by experimental embryologists. Large graft exchanges made for a variety of experimental purposes have frequently shown remarkable survival of the resulting chimaeras. Figure 5.1 illustrates some of the manipulative procedures which can produce immunological tolerance. Even after extreme surgical inter-

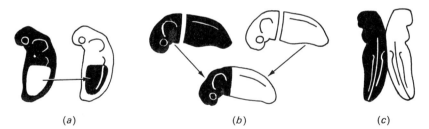

(a)   (b)   (c)

Figure 5.1. Embryonic microsurgery and tolerance induction in urodeles

Some of the microsurgical procedures which can lead to tolerance induction when performed on 2–3 mm urodele embryos at the tail-bud stage of development are illustrated.

(a) Large grafts of flank integument transplanted orthotopically.

(b) Transection of the embryo and fusion of the anterior half of one embryo to the posterior half of another embryo.

(c) Joining together two embryos side by side (parabiosis).

From Houillon, C. (1972), "Les réactions immunitaires chez les amphibiens urodèles. II. Interventions microchirurgicales sur les embryons", pp. 97–104 in *L'etude phylogénique et ontogénique de la réponse immunitaire et son apport à la théorie immunologique*, Société Française d'Immunologie Symposium, Paris (with modifications).

vention (e.g. when anterior and posterior halves of the embryo are exchanged) survival times of several years have been recorded—up to 8 years in allogeneic chimaeras of the Spanish newt *Pleurodeles waltlii*. Life-long chimaeras can also be obtained by joining embryos of the same species side by side in parabiotic union. Even in some xenogeneic combinations good survival has been recorded. Tolerance is not necessarily the outcome however: some inter-species combinations are incompatible and some grafts (e.g. embryonic ectodermal grafts from *P. waltlii* placed on axolotl embryos) are in fact rejected after a period of several months, presumably when the immune system of the host larva becomes sufficiently mature.

Experiments on allogeneic chimaeras formed by joining half embryos indicate that each half of the chimaera retains its own particular antigenicity. Thus grafts taken from the anterior half and those from the posterior half of the chimaera may be rejected at different times when transplanted onto a third-party host. The continued presence of two incompatible cellular populations can lead in some cases (particularly in xenogeneic combinations) to a runting disease from which the animal eventually dies. For example, when *P. waltlii* is joined in embryonic parabiosis with either *T. alpestris* or the palmate newt *T. helveticus*, runting eventually sets in after about 3 to 5 months. This is probably due to a graft-versus-host reaction in which immunologically competent graft cells attack the tissues of the host. Runting has also been recorded in adult Japanese newts joined tail to tail in allogeneic combinations.

Despite these exceptions, tolerance induction in general is easily achieved in urodeles, and graft-versus-host reactions are relatively weak. Furthermore allogeneic organ grafts (such as those of heart or gonads) often survive for long periods with no obvious signs of immune attack, even in animals hyperimmunized with skin grafts. This is consistent with the lack of strong histocompatibility barriers, tolerance being more readily attained when only weak disparaties are present.

5.1.3. *"In vitro" responses*

Lymphocytes from urodeles respond less well than those from anuran amphibians when cultured *in vitro* with phytohaemagglutinin (PHA). Furthermore, no obvious stimulation has yet been demonstrated in mixed lymphocyte cultures in urodeles. It is unlikely that this poor mitogenic response to allogeneic histocompatibility antigens in the mixed lymphocyte reaction is due to lack of proper culture conditions, since anuran (frog) lymphocytes consistently show strong stimulation when used in parallel experiments. There seems to be a genuine difference between urodeles and anurans in their mixed lymphocyte reactivity, and this difference may well relate to the lack of a major histocompatibility complex in the former group.

5.1.4. *Antibody production*

Structural details on urodele immunoglobulins are as yet relatively limited, but it appears that in urodeles, only one class of antibody (IgM) is produced. Where low-molecular-weight antibody has been detected, e.g. in axolotls immunized with a bacteriophage, this antibody comprises quickly sedimenting IgM subunits with a μ-type heavy chain. These low-molecular-weight antibodies, like the high-molecular-weight IgM, are sensitive to inhibition by 2-mercaptoethanol.

Axolotls give good but delayed antibody production to bacterial antigens, such as *Salmonella typhimurium*, *S. typhosa* and *Brucella abortus*, and to bacteriophages, but they fail to respond to soluble antigens (pig serum and ferritin). Soluble antigens are usually also poor immunogens in *P. waltlii* and *T. alpestris*, although these newts show positive antibody responses to haemocyanin (a soluble antigen of high molecular weight), as well as to *S. typhimurium*, *B. abortus* and sheep erythrocytes. Axolotls have been immunized both as larvae and in the adult state. The antibody response is essentially similar in the two forms.

When axolotls *Ambystoma mexicanum* and Spanish newts *P. waltlii* were immunized with *B. abortus* at temperatures of 20 °C and 26 °C respectively, agglutinating antibody was detected in the serum in the second to third week after injection of the antigen, and rose to its maximum value at 50–100 days. Secondary immunization in the 5th month yielded a further modest increase in the titre. Even one year after immunization the serum antibody was still all of high molecular weight; most was sensitive to inhibition by 2-mercaptoethanol, although some of the high-molecular-weight antibody was 2-mercaptoethanol-resistant.

Cellular co-operation in antibody production has been demonstrated in the common American (red spotted) newt. These studies were the first to demonstrate such co-operation in a poikilotherm. It is now believed to occur also in anurans and in teleost fish, and probably represents an early and fundamental aspect of antibody production in vertebrates. In the experiments on the common American newt, the hapten-carrier system comprised trinitrophenol (TNP) coupled to erythrocytes, and the response was measured using immunocytoadherence tests (see figure 4.2). It was found that preimmunization with the carrier erythrocytes, followed four days later by injection of carrier coupled with hapten, led to the appearance of cells capable of forming rosettes with anti-hapten (TNP) specificity. These rosette-forming cells (RFC) occurred amongst the lymphoid populations of spleen, liver and kidney. In order to elicit this reaction, the foreign erythrocytes initially used to preimmunize the newt had to be the same as those coupled with the TNP. For example, if chicken erythrocytes were used for preimmunization, chicken (and not toad) erythrocytes had to be coupled with TNP for the second injection. The co-operation of at least two populations of immunologically competent cells is indicated by these experiments—one population specific for the carrier which helps another population to generate its anti-hapten response. By analogy with mammalian studies on cellular co-operation in antibody formation (see Chapter 1, p. 28), we might expect the carrier specificity to reside in a T-cell population, but this has yet to be established for any poikilotherm.

5.1.5. *Lymphoid tissues*

Histogenesis and functional development of the thymus

In the Apoda, a primitive branchiomeric arrangement of the thymic anlagen is retained. Epithelial buds develop dorsally in relation to each pair of pharyngeal pouches, including those of the spiracular region. Of these, the first and last atrophy, and the remaining four pairs undergo thymic histogenesis to produce four pairs of definitive thymic nodules.

In the embryos of urodeles there may initially be five pairs of thymic buds, of which two soon disappear, leaving those from pouches 3, 4 and 5 to differentiate and form the thymus (see figure 4.1). This isolates as a three-lobed organ in the connective tissue behind the mandible. In some newts, however, the thymus is formed entirely by the 5th pouch, and the existence of anlagen associated with any of the other pharyngeal regions is doubtful. Thymic differentiation appears to involve entry of mesen-chymatous cells into the developing organ. In the thymus of adult urodeles the distinction between cortex and medulla is less marked than in the majority of vertebrates.

In urodeles the immune system differentiates only slowly. For example, in *T. alpestris* the thymus does not develop until the 7th week of life. As in all vertebrates, histogenesis of the secondary lymphoid organs occurs after that of the thymus, and in *T. alpestris* differentiation of the spleen commences at week 9. The maturation of cell-mediated immuno-competence is a correspondingly leisurely process. Axolotls reared at 21 °C did not respond effectively to skin allografts until they were about three months old; likewise, their ability to bring about regression of histoincompatible tumours also developed at about this time. Another factor of importance in larval transplantation studies concerns the histo-compatibility antigens themselves; these also show a gradual increase in their abilities to elicit rejection during the course of development.

Effect of thymectomy

Animals which possess free-living larval stages provide excellent models for investigation of the role of the primary lymphoid organs. Thus in amphibian larvae, for example, the thymus can be removed at a much earlier stage of development than is technically feasible in an amniote. Larvae in which the thymic buds derive from a single pair of pharyngeal pouches (rather than from several pairs, see figure 4.1*c*) have proved particularly suitable for use in these experiments. Such larvae include those of anuran amphibians (section 6.1.5) and those of some newts (e.g. *Pleurodeles* and *Triturus*).

In *P. waltlii*, *T. alpestris* and in the tiger salamander *Ambystoma tigrinum*, thymectomy abolishes or significantly delays the rejection of skin allografts. In these experiments the thymectomized animals usually remained in good health, although some succumbed after a year or more to a wasting disease resembling that described in thymectomized mice. In *P. waltlii* the thymus was only 300–450 μm in diameter when it was removed at the age of 8 weeks; in *T. alpestris* it was removed at week 10. In *T. alpestris* the splenic RFC (rosette-forming cell) response to sheep erythrocytes was examined as well as the allograft reactivity; both were found to be suppressed after early thymectomy.

Other lymphoid tissues

In comparison with anuran amphibians, the organization of the lymphoid organs in urodeles shows little or no advance over that of the fishes. The main lymphoid organs are the thymus and spleen. There are no lymph nodes in urodeles, and there is no well-organized gut-associated lymphoid tissue. The bone marrow is not a haemopoietic tissue except in some members of the Family Plethodontidae (lungless salamanders). The intertubular tissue of the kidney and the subcapsular layer of the liver take part in blood-cell formation. Their role is mainly to provide granulocytes, but lymphoid tissue also occurs in these areas in some urodeles. In the giant Japanese salamander, the meningeal region in the head is a site where lymphocytes are produced. The spleen is the principal secondary lymphoid organ in urodeles. It develops as a collection of mesenchymatous cells in association with the splenic blood vessels. As in other vertebrates, its lymphoid tissue accompanies the arterial vasculature, but it is not clearly demarcated into well-defined white-pulp and red-pulp areas. Plasma cells have been described in the lamina propria of the gut, but they are not usually present in great numbers, either in this region or elsewhere in the body in urodeles.

A number of experiments clearly demonstrate the immunocompetence of lymphocytes of the spleen, liver and kidney. Allogeneic spleen cells (and to a lesser extent liver cells) have been shown to elicit a form of graft-verses-host disease when transferred into immunologically deficient (irradiated) Japanese newts, and similar cells of autologous (self) origin can restore alloimmune reactivity to such hosts. Cells which form rosettes with sheep erythrocytes (RFC) have been demonstrated in the spleens of *P. waltlii* and *T. alpestris* following immunization with this antigen. In the common American newt, *N. viridescens*, comparisons have been made of RFCs in spleen, liver and kidney when the newts were injected with horse erythrocytes. Cells forming rosettes with horse erythrocytes were found in all three tissues, with higher numbers in the spleen than in the liver or kidney. In spleen and kidney the numbers of RFC were higher in secondary responses than in the primary response. Results from splenectomized animals yielded data which suggest that in the primary response the RFCs are generated *in situ*, but in the secondary response there may be lymphoid-cell traffic between spleen and liver.

Apart from these findings, very little effect of splenectomy upon the immune response has been reported for urodeles. In *N. viridescens*, splenectomy failed to prolong allograft survival, while in *P. waltlii* very early removal of the spleen at a time when it starts to develop did not affect growth of the animal or its susceptibility to infections and, again, allografts were rejected normally.

5.2. Conclusions

In general it would appear that with respect to their immunobiology, as well as with other aspects of their anatomy and physiology, the urodeles (and possibly also the apodans) remain close to the condition of their fish-like ancestors. In the slow rejection of allografts, the restriction of antibody synthesis to μ-chain (IgM) immunoglobulins and in the relative simplicity of their lymphoid organs, these amphibians are in marked contrast to the more advanced anurans. Although some urodeles are terrestrial as adults, there is a general tendency in the group to persist as aquatic animals, and a number of types never leave the water. In their immune system also, they should perhaps be regarded as an evolutionarily conservative group.

CHAPTER SIX

EMERGENCE ON TO LAND:
THE AMPHIBIANS—ANURA

6.1. Anura

The fossil record of anurans dates from the Triassic period, but there is little indication of when they diverged from the other modern amphibian groups. A major specialization during anuran evolution has been the exploitation of two distinct phases in the life history: an aquatic herbivorous stage and a more terrestrial (and more carnivorous) adult. This specialization which is developed to a greater extreme in anurans than in urodele amphibians, probably relates historically to the periodic availability of water, the prolonged larval stage being an adaptation which allowed the larvae to remain in, and exploit, rich feeding grounds available during the wet season.

The anuran tadpole is clearly an immature animal, since it is neither fully grown nor sexually developed. At the same time its prolonged immaturity is itself a specialization, and a reasonable level of efficiency in the defence mechanisms at this stage is only to be expected. The marked change in body form between the larva and adult, and the rapid anatomical and biochemical reorganization which accompanies anuran metamorphosis, have immunological implications which will be discussed later in this chapter.

In addition to their use for ontogenetic studies, amphibians are of obvious interest as modern descendants of the early tetrapods, representing as they do a transitional stage in the move from an aquatic to a terrestrial habit.

6.1.1. *Transplantation reactions*

The more advanced anurans such as those of the families Ranidae (the ranid frogs) and Bufonidae (the bufid toads) show acute rejection of histoincompatible grafts. For example, in the bullfrog *Rana catesbeiana*, first-set skin allografts are rejected within two weeks at 25 °C. At the histological level, the sequence of graft rejection is essentially similar to that in urodeles (capillary dilation with haemostasis and breakdown, lymphocytic infiltration, disintegration of pigment cells and death of the epithelial and glandular components of the graft) but in anurans these events take place more rapidly. Accelerated second-set responses occur regularly; indeed in advanced anurans second-set grafts rarely become vascularized.

In more primitive anurans of the families Pipidae, e.g. the clawed toad *Xenopus laevis* (figure 6.1) and Discoglossidae (e.g. the midwife toad *Alytes obstetricans*) rejection is a somewhat more prolonged process. In *X. laevis* the response to first-set allografts takes about three weeks at 23 °C. Similarly, in *A. obstetricans*, rejection times of between 21 and 33 days have been recorded. Second-set grafts are usually rejected more rapidly than first-set grafts; in *X. laevis* they may or may not become revascularized before they are rejected. Some of the variability can be attributed to different degrees of antigen-sharing in laboratory colonies; nevertheless the subacute rejection times and the prolonged survival of grafts on some animals place these primitive anurans in a position intermediate between the urodeles and the more advanced frogs and toads.

Temperature has a marked effect on alloimmune responses in *X. laevis*. In animals kept at 9 °C the rejection of first-set skin allografts takes over 200 days. The second-set response is affected to a lesser extent, rejection times being 33 days at 9 °C compared with 8 days at 25 °C. This is similar to urodeles: in newts, the delaying effect of low temperatures is greater in first-set than in second-set responses.

6.1.2. *Ontogeny of transplantation reactivity*

Onset of immunocompetence

Clear-cut alloimmune responses occur in larvae as well as in adult anurans. In *R. catesbeiana* the ability to recognize and destroy skin allografts develops at the time when small lymphocytes first appear in the blood. Similarly in *X. laevis* larvae, the first indications of reactivity can be correlated with the state of differentiation of the lymphoid tissues. The thymus is the first lymphoid organ to develop, and once thymic histogenesis has reached the stage when small lymphocytes are present in the organ, the larva becomes capable of making a lymphocytic response to an allograft.

If grafts are placed on very young larvae whose lymphoid organs are immature at the time of application, lymphocytic invasion of the graft is delayed, but it eventually occurs when the host reaches a more advanced stage of differentiation. Skin grafts placed on 5-day old *X. laevis* larvae eventually succumb to immunological attack as the host matures. Also, in even earlier transplantation experiments, it has been shown that tail-tip allografts transplanted into embryos of the leopard frog *Rana pipiens* eventually elicit a lymphocytic response; so also does embryologically

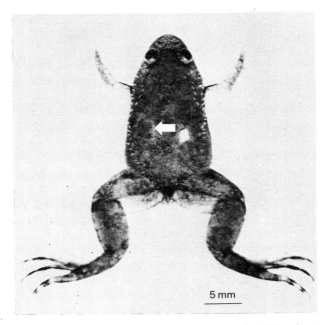

5 mm

Figure 6.1 shows a young clawed toad (*Xenopus laevis*) bearing two skin grafts. On the left side of the back is an autograft, i.e. a transplant of the animal's own skin; on the right is an allograft, i.e. skin from another individual of the same species. The photograph was taken three weeks after the grafts were applied. The animal shows no immune response to the autograft; this has healed in well and is barely discernible (an arrow marks its medial edge). The allograft appears white owing to disintegration of its pigment cells, and destruction of the epithelial and glandular components. Allograft rejection is well advanced in this animal.

From Horton, J. D. (1969), "Ontogeny of the Immune Response to Skin Allografts in relation to Lymphoid Organ Development in the Amphibian *Xenopus laevis* Daudin", *Journal of Experimental Zoology*, **170**, 449–466.

grafted neural fold material. Hence early exposure to a foreign antigen does not necessarily preclude the possibility of an immune response to the same antigen in the more mature animal. This is not unexpected: a free-living larva will encounter pathogens in its environment before its lymphoid system is mature enough to deal with them. In the young larva the first line of defence is probably the phagocytic system; thus in X. *laevis* free macrophages have been shown to function at a very early stage in development before the lymphocytic system has matured.

Ontogeny of histocompatibility antigens

As in other poikilotherms (see, for example, section 4.2.1) histo-compatibility antigens can be demonstrated in the embryo. Thus X. *laevis* embryos implanted into a sensitized host elicited a second-set response. In these experiments sensitization of the recipient was achieved by obtaining a first-set response to a maternal skin graft (from the embryo's parent) before implanting the embryonic tissue. The subsequent second-set response to the embryonic implant indicated that the main histo-compatibility antigens were already present in the embryo. It has also been shown that grafts of embryonic tissue can sensitize a host, so that later on it gives second-set reactions to skin grafts from the same donor.

Additional new antigens appear as differentiation proceeds and cells start to make their own specific products. The animal normally becomes tolerant of these organ-specific transplantation antigens; their presence can, however, be demonstrated experimentally. Thus in the tree frog *Hyla regilla*, antigens associated with the hypophysis were demonstrated by removing the buccal component of the pituitary gland at an embryonic stage, growing it in another individual, and then grafting it back to its original owner. The hypophyseal graft was rejected because, during its residence in the temporary recipient, new organ-specific (hypophyseal) antigens had developed which had not been encountered by the original owner and which were not recognized as "self".

Events at metamorphosis

The anatomical and biochemical modifications which accompany anuran metamorphosis are more extreme than in most other vertebrates, and therefore exaggerate the immunological problems associated with the acquisition of new antigens. Indeed, there are strong indications that there is a partial suppression of the immune response as the animal changes from one form to another. Thus in *X. laevis* the ability to reject skin grafts from siblings is much impaired around the time of metamorphosis, and the animals apparently become tolerant to certain histocompatibility antigens. Indeed, when large grafts are exchanged between siblings during metamorphosis, 75% are tolerated (compared with 25% tolerance of small grafts). Possibly, for these large grafts a single haplotype difference does not suffice to provoke a histocompatibility reaction. Since the major histocompatibility locus appears to be operationally rather weak in *X. laevis*, it may require a two-haplotype difference to bring about large-graft rejection during the perimetamorphic period.

During metamorphosis, changes occur in the thymus. Thus there is a temporary decrease in the total number of cells in the organ, and a fall in the percentage of thymic lymphocytes expressing immunoglobulin on their surface; possibly thymic function is suppressed during this critical period. The blood-serum proteins increase in concentration with the move to a terrestrial environment, and during metamorphosis there is a rise in serum albumin and a relative decrease in globulins; this is accompanied by a temporary fall in antibody titres.

Tolerance induction

In anurans, as in other vertebrates, tolerance to implanted tissues can be induced experimentally (see figure 6.2). The outcome of embryonic exposure to allografts (whether the animal becomes tolerant or whether an immune response is elicited) depends on the size of the graft. Apparently, the host's reactive system can only be suppressed by a large amount of transplanted material. Thus large tail-tip allografts applied to *R. pipiens* embryos induce a permanent state of tolerance, but small tail-tip allografts are rejected. Similarly, a large amount of neural fold material is tolerated, whereas immunity ensues when small grafts are used (figure 6.3). In *X. laevis* a massive graft taken from the flank of an embryo at the neurula stage of development induces specific tolerance when transferred ortho-topically to another neurula. In this situation a graft-versus-host reaction can be induced later in life. Thus if, as a young toad, the donor is sensitized to the recipient by means of skin grafts, and the spleen from this sensitized animal is then transferred into the recipient, a marked inflammatory response ensues as the immunologically competent spleen cells attack the tolerant host.

Embryonic parabiosis in anurans is usually successful only in allogeneic combinations; in these a state of tolerance is induced. The parabionts are,

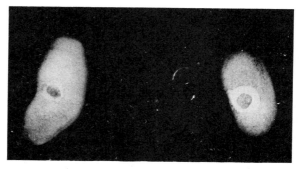

1 mm

Figure 6.2 shows two early embryos of the amphibian *Xenopus laevis*, photographed shortly after the exchange of grafts from one embryo to the other. The operation is performed on the day after fertilization. The jelly coats and vitelline membrane are removed, and the embryo is placed into a well cut in blackened agar. The graft is held in place by a piece of glass coverslip, the edges of which can be seen in the photograph. At this stage in the procedure the grafts have contracted and no longer cover the graft bed. They heal in rapidly, however, and the embryos soon recover their normal appearance. In sibling embryos from the same spawning (as pictured here), grafts of this size induce mutual specific tolerance of the partner's tissues.
  Courtesy of Mrs. Andrea Randall of the University of Hull.

in fact, chimaeras in the sense that they each carry blood cells which properly belong to their partner. This has been demonstrated in *R. pipiens*, a species in which triploid embryos can be produced using a technique of pressure treatment to the ovulated egg. When these triploid embryos are joined to normal diploid forms, their cells can be traced to the partner. After separation of the parabionts the foreign cells persist. Their presence apparently promotes the state of tolerance, but this wanes after separation, and their numbers decline as new immunologically competent cells emerge from within the host.

6.1.3. *"In vitro" responses*

Lymphocytes taken from *X. laevis*, as well as those from more advanced anurans (e.g. the marine toad *Bufo marinus*) readily respond to stimulation *in vitro*. This has been demonstrated using non-specific mitogens such as phytohaemagglutinin (PHA), and in mixed lymphocyte culture (MLC). Family studies in *X. laevis* suggest that genetic control of MLC reactivity in anurans is essentially similar to that in mammals. Thus when thymus cells from sibships (brothers and sisters) of known parentage were tested in all possible pairs within their own sibship and with unrelated individuals, data on the level of stimulation obtained in each combination clearly indicate control by a single genetic region. There is also a well-defined haplotype effect whereby the MLC reaction is approximately half as strong when the individuals differ by only one haplotype (one allele of the pair) than when there is a two-haplotype difference.

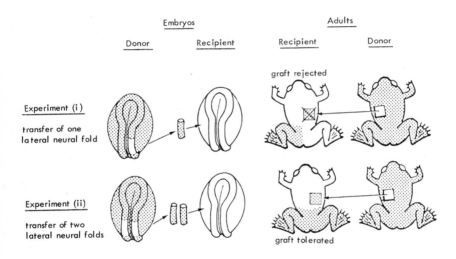

Figure 6.3. Dosage effect in the induction of tolerance to allografts
Experiments on the leopard frog *Rana pipiens*, in which lateral neural folds from one embryo are grafted onto another embryo of the same age, are illustrated.
In experiment (i) only one lateral fold is transferred. This fails to induce tolerance in the recipient and a subsequent graft of skin taken from the same donor and applied to the host frog after metamorphosis is rejected. In experiment (ii), in contrast, both lateral folds are transferred and this larger "double dose" renders the recipient specifically tolerant to subsequent allografts taken from the same donor.
From Volpe, E. P. (1972), "Embryonic Tissue Transplantation Incompatibility in an Amphibian", *American Scientist*, **60**, 220–228 (with modifications).

6.1.4. *Humoral immunity in Anura*

Immunoglobulin classes

Two classes of immunoglobulin can be detected in the serum of anuran amphibians. These proteins are antigenically distinct; their heavy chains have different molecular weights, and they show different electrophoretic mobilities on immunoelectrophoresis. They have been tentatively classified as IgM and IgG because of their general resemblance to the IgM and IgG immunoglobulins of mammals. The two classes occur in tadpoles, as well as in adult anurans. The molecular weight of the IgM is consistent with a pentameric structure. However, in *X. laevis*, a hexameric (six sub-unit) form has been revealed by electron microscopy.

The anuran low-molecular-weight immunoglobulin resembles mammalian IgG and, if homologous, represents the first appearance of IgG in vertebrates. Much of the evidence based on physicochemical properties suggests that its heavy chains (γ-chains) are indeed similar to those of mammals. However, certain differences in electrophoretic mobility between the γ-chains of mammalian IgG and those of the low-molecular-weight immunoglobulin obtained from *R. catesbeiana* or from *X. laevis*, indicate some structural variation. More information is required before the significance of these findings can be interpreted but, in any event, the anurans show a clear advance when compared with urodeles in the diversity of their immunoglobulin classes; they can synthesize both IgM and IgG-like immunoglobulins, whereas in urodeles, and in most fishes, only a single class (IgM) is produced.

Antibody production

Although both IgM and IgG-like antibodies are produced by anurans, the IgG seems to play a less prominent role than in mammals. Indeed with particulate antigens such as bacteria and foreign erythrocytes, IgM may be the only antibody synthesized. Bacteriophages and soluble foreign proteins regularly elicit both IgM and IgG production, but even in these responses the IgG is slow to appear by mammalian standards, and it only partially replaces IgM during the time course of the response. Thus, when marine toads *B. marinus* are immunized with bacteriophage at 22 °C and their serum tested for the presence of neutralizing antibody, activity is detected only in the IgM class for the first month after immunization, although in the second month IgG-like antibody begins to supplement the IgM production. In non-immunized clawed toads *X. laevis*, the amount of low-molecular-weight immunoglobulin in the serum is variable and may be quite low. IgG-like antibody has been elicited in *X. laevis* by protozoan antigens (*Tetrahymena pyriformis*) as well as by foreign serum proteins. Again the first antibody to be produced is IgM,

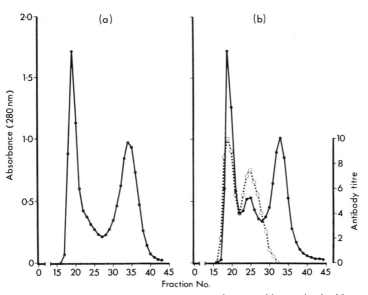

serum from non-immunized toad

serum from toad immunized with
human gamma globulin (HGG) in adjuvant

Figure 6.4.   Gel filtration on Sephadex G-200 of normal and immune
Xenopus **serum**

(a) Diagram (a) shows the profile obtained for serum proteins of normal *Xenopus laevis*. The first (higher) peak contains IgM immunoglobulin. The other peak is albumin.

(b) After immunization with human gamma globulin (HGG) in Freund's complete adjuvant, anti-HGG antibodies appear in the serum (dotted line). By the second month these are distributed in two distinct peaks. The heavier (IgM) immunoglobulin is the first to appear in the elution profile (on the left); this antibody is 2-mercaptoethanol-sensitive. The low-molecular-weight (IgG-like) antibody in the second peak is 2-mercaptoethanol-resistant and shows precipitating activity against HGG.

From Manning, M. J. (1975), "The Phylogeny of Thymic Dependence", *American Zoologist*, **15**, 63–71. See also, Turner, R. J. and Manning, M. J. (1974), "Thymic Dependence of Amphibian Antibody Responses", *European Journal of Immunology*, **4**, 343–346.

detectable mainly by tests involving haemagglutinating and haemolytic activity; this antibody is 2-mercaptoethanol-sensitive. The later antibody is the low-molecular-weight IgG form which is efficient in precipitating soluble antigens and which is 2-mercaptoethanol-resistant (see figure 6.4).

Amphibians apparently lack the capacity for immunological memory to antigens such as the bacterial flagellar antigens of *Salmonella adelaide* which elicit purely IgM responses. This largely holds for antibody production to foreign erythrocytes, where serum antibody is produced more quickly on secondary challenge but not in appreciably higher amounts, and the response remains that of IgM production. Enhanced secondary responses are more evident after immunization with antigens which evoke low-molecular-weight antibody. For example, *B. marinus* shows immunological memory on secondary stimulation with bacteriophage or with bovine serum albumin (BSA). This includes a reduction of the latent period before antibody appears in the circulation, a more rapid rise in antibody titre, a longer-lasting peak response, and an increase in the IgG to IgM ratio. Negative memory, as well as positive immunity, can be induced by this type of antigen. This has been demonstrated in *B. marinus*, where specific tolerance to BSA was elicited following injection of high doses of antigen in amounts similar to those which induce tolerance in mammals. A relationship between clearly defined secondary responses and IgG production is well known for mammals, but in amphibians a wider range of antigens appear to elicit a purely IgM response with little or no memory component.

One difficulty in studying the secondary responses to soluble antigens in amphibians is that antigen from the first injection may well persist in the circulation for many months (figure 6.5). It is therefore necessary to distinguish secondary responses from the effects of increased antigen dose on an on-going primary response. Another characteristic of antibody production to soluble antigens in this group is the high requirement for substances known as *adjuvants*. This is particularly marked in the more primitive anurans. Indeed, *X. laevis* rarely responds to foreign serum proteins if these are administered on their own, whereas good antibody responses are obtained when the antigen is mixed with adjuvant before injection. Freund's complete adjuvant, a water-in-oil emulsion containing killed tubercle bacilli, is often used. In mammals this adjuvant is believed to increase antibody production, partly by acting as a depot, partly by stimulating phagocytosis, and partly as a consequence of cell-mediated responses evoked through sensitized T-cells. In amphibians, assistance in localizing and trapping the antigen may be very important in animals not

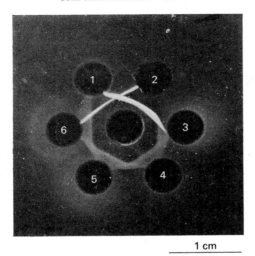

1 cm

Figure 6.5 shows the technique of double diffusion in agar (the Ouchterlony method) in which antibody is placed in a central well cut in agar gel and antigen is placed in peripheral wells. Antibody and antigen diffuse towards each other in the gel to form an opaque white line of precipitation in the region where they meet in optimal proportions.

In the Ouchterlony plate photographed here, the central well was filled with an antibody to whole human serum, peripheral well 1 contained one of the components of human serum (its gamma globulin fraction), while well 2 contained another component (human serum albumin). A strong white line of precipitation has developed between the antibody which was placed in the central well and the human gamma globulin placed in well 1. There is also a strong line between the central well and well 2, formed by precipitation of the albumin fraction.

In this experiment toads (*Xenopus laevis*) were injected with whole human serum and tested four weeks later for persistence of foreign protein in their circulation. Samples of their serum were placed in wells 3, 4, 5 and 6. The white line between these wells and the central well shows that some of the antigen (human serum) was still present in the toad serum. Furthermore, it indicates that human serum ablumin, but not the gamma globulin fraction, was persisting. This can be deduced from the fact that the line of precipitation of antigen from the toads' serum is confluent with that from the albumin in well 2 (indicating antigenic identity with the human albumin) but it crosses the line formed by precipitation of human gamma globulin (between wells 1 and 6), indicating non-identity with the gamma globulin fraction of human serum.

From Turner, R. J. (1974), "Effects of Splenectomy on Amphibian Antibody Responses", *Experientia*, **30**, 1089–1090.

otherwise well equipped for dealing with non-particulate material, and the high requirement for adjuvant when soluble antigens are used could reflect a lack of sophistication in the antigen-trapping mechanisms, especially in species such as *X. laevis* which have no lymph nodes.

Effects of temperature

Poikilotherms might be expected to give a good level of immunological reactivity at the temperature at which they normally live, and to be less efficient at sub-optimal temperatures. Their body temperature will frequently be below that of mammals. However, any relative slowness or deficiencies in their humoral responses cannot be attributed entirely to this cause. Tropical amphibians can be kept successfully at 37 °C and, in *B. marinus* for example, vigorous responses are obtained to *Salmonella adelaide* flagellae at this temperature—nevertheless, the toads still fail to show immunological memory to the bacterial antigen.

Such susceptibility of immune reactivity to environmental temperature makes the amphibians a useful experimental model for investigating the effect of temperature on the different stages of immune reactions, and a number of experiments have been performed in which animals are moved from one temperature to another during various parts of the response. From these it appears that in amphibians, as in fishes, only certain stages are temperature-dependent: the initial event of antigen recognition occurs irrespective of whether the animal is kept at high or low temperature, and it is the second step, resulting in antibody production, which is more dependent on suitable temperature conditions. Thus, in *B. marinus* injected with foreign (horse) erythrocytes, there was no appreciable difference between the numbers of splenic lymphocytes forming specific rosettes (RFC) at 20 °C and at 37 °C in the early part of the response (at day 3). However, from day 3 to day 6, the temperature was important in determining both the number of RFC present at day 6 and the appearance of circulating antibody. In experiments on marine toads immunized with bacteriophage and transferred from 25 °C to 15 °C at a later stage in the response (after 2 weeks), the serum antibody levels were only temporarily depressed, although there was a marked delay in the conversion from high-molecular-weight to low-molecular-weight antibodies. Release of antibody at low temperature and the maintenance of serum antibody levels may have an adaptive significance in relation to disease resistance during cold periods in amphibians, similar to that already discussed in fish (see section 4.2.3).

Immediate hypersensitivity reactions

There are very few studies on immediate hypersensitivity reactions in poikilotherms. However, in leopard frogs *R. pipiens* immunized with *Salmonella typhosa* vaccine, a subsequent challenge with soluble antigen from the corresponding bacteria (*S. typhosa*) led to shock symptoms with a flaccid paralysis which was fatal in two cases. These symptoms were similar to those of histamine shock and suggest that an immune reaction of the immediate hypersensitivity type had occurred, perhaps mediated through the amphibian low-molecular-weight antibody.

Ontogeny of antibody synthesis

Since the early developmental stages of amphibians are readily accessible, these animals can be immunized at an age when their lymphoid system contains only small numbers of cells. Larvae of the midwife toad *Alytes obstetricans*, injected with foreign erythrocytes at a time when the total number of lymphocytes in the body was less than one million, were able to respond with the appearance of specific plaque-forming cells (PFC) and rosette-forming cells (RFC) in their spleens. These larvae were usually less than two months old, and their splenic lymphocytes numbered between 6,000 and 15,000 cells. Similarly tadpoles of *Rana catesbeiana* could respond to DNP (dinitrophenol)- and TNP (trinitrophenol)-conjugated bacteria and proteins at an age when they possessed a total of about two million lymphocytes. Furthermore, the tadpoles were able to discriminate between these structurally similar determinants and to produce hapten-specific non-cross-reacting anti-DNP and anti-TNP antibodies. Thus the specificity of antibodies produced by these small larvae appears to be equivalent to that of older and larger animals and, indeed, to rival mammalian capabilities. A similar situation obtains for cell-mediated allograft responses in *X. laevis* larvae, where specific lymphocytic reactions to grafts can occur when the larvae have less than one million lymphocytes in the body.

These findings have important implications for theories of the origin of antibody diversity, since numerically there are insufficient lymphocytes present rigidly to fulfil the requirements of the clonal selection theory (see figure 1.4). Perhaps some lymphocytes are multipotential with regard to their receptor sites, or possibly some diversity may arise during the course of antigen-driven proliferation.

Non-immunoglobulin factors and complement

Natural defence factors which are not immunoglobulins occur in amphibians as in other vertebrates. In *Alytes obstetricans*, a non-immunoglobulin cytolytic factor can be demonstrated. This does not depend on complement for its activity and is lipoprotein in nature.

The serum complement systems of amphibians (urodeles and anurans) have components similar to those of mammals, and they show a close similarity in dose response studies. However, frog complement reacts more effectively at 16 °C than at 37 °C, even when substituted for mammalian complement in a mammalian haemolytic system (i.e. using mammalian antibody).

6.1.5. *Lymphoid tissues*

Anurans show a considerable advance in comparison with urodeles in the possession of a haemopoietic bone marrow, well-organized nodules of lymphoid tissue in the gastro-intestinal tract and, in ranid frogs and bufid toads, rudimentary lymph nodes. Table 6.1 shows the major lymphoid organs of larval and adult *X. laevis*. In the more advanced

Table 6.1. Major lymphoid organs of the amphibian *Xenopus laevis*

Larva	Adult
thymus	thymus
spleen	spleen
pharyngeal ventral cavity bodies	lymphoid tissue of gut (mainly intestinal)
lymphoid tissue of the kidney (mesonephros)	lymphoid tissue of the kidney (mesonephros)
lymphoid tissue of the liver (mainly subcapsular)	lymphoid tissue of the liver (mainly subcapsular)
	a few lymphocytic accumulations in the skin
	bone marrow

Xenopus laevis lacks the larval lymph glands and the adult lymph nodes which are found in more advanced anurans.

anurans, larval lymph glands and adult lymph nodes are added. Some lymphoid organs, such as the thymus and spleen, retain their integrity from larva to adult, but others are involved in the profound changes which affect the branchial apparatus, gut and skeletal elements at metamorphosis. Thus the pharyngeal lymphocytic accumulations of the larva (the ventral cavity bodies—see figure 6.6) which lie in a sentinel position in relation to the larval exhalent water current, disappear at metamorphosis when the branchial apparatus is lost; well-defined gut-associated lymphoid nodules develop as the gut undergoes extensive reorganization and acquires its adult form; bone marrow appears as the cartilaginous skeleton of the larva gives rise to adult bones; while the definitive lymph nodes of the advanced anurans appear near the beginning of metamorphosis, and increase in size in the developing throat and axillary region of the adult as the larval lymph gland shrinks and disappears.

Development of the Thymus

The paired thymus in anurans arises as a dorsal bud from the left and right second pharyngeal pouch (see figure 1.11 and figure 4.1c); it is the

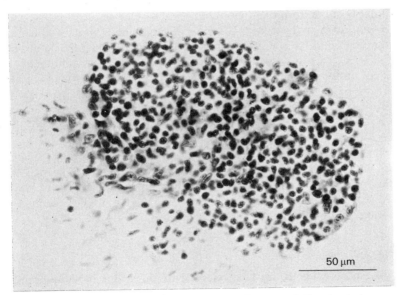

50 μm

Figure 6.6 shows a pharyngeal lymphocytic accumulation (ventral cavity body) of a *Xenopus laevis* larva. The majority of the cells in this simple lymphoid organ are small lymphocytes with their rounded deeply-stained nuclei. Ventral cavity bodies are situated in sentinel positions in relation to the openings of the branchial chambers. The subepithelial lymphocytes lie close to the pharyngeal lumen; they are separated from it by a single layer of attenuated epithelial cells.

From Manning, M. J. and Horton, J. D. (1969), "Histogenesis of Lymphoid Organs in Larvae of the South African Clawed Toad, *Xenopus laevis* (Daudin)", *Journal of Embryology and Experimental Morphology*, **22**, 265–277.

first lymphoid organ to develop. Recent experiments, in which thymus cells were labelled and traced at a very early stage in thymic differentiation, demonstrate that thymic lymphocytes arise *in situ* from the presumptive thymic rudiment, and that virtually all lymphocytes in the spleen, kidneys and bone marrow also originate from this source. These experiments were done with leopard frogs *Rana pipiens* using a triploid donor frog produced by pressure treatment of the ovulated egg. The presumptive thymic area of the 72-hour-old donor was placed orthotopically onto a diploid embryo of the same age whose own thymus area had been removed. The *in situ* origin of thymic lymphocytes in *R. pipiens* contrasts with findings in avian and mammalian studies (discussed in Chapter 8, section 8.1.7). The nature of the stem cells in the anuran experiments is unknown. They evidently arise within the transplanted tissue and presumably come from the thymic rudiment itself.

The anuran thymus consists of a pair of single-lobed organs which are clearly differentiated into cortex and medulla (see figure 6.7). In anuran amphibians as in fish (section 4.2.5), surface immunoglobulins can be detected on thymic lymphocytes and can be shown to be synthesized by these cells. In *X. laevis* the thymus is the first source of lymphocytes bearing detectable surface-associated immunoglobulin. These appear at a time before the spleen is populated with lymphocytes, at about one week after fertilization. Throughout larval life and up to one month after metamorphosis, the percentage of immunoglobulin-bearing cells in the thymus is high (up to 80% compared with approximately 50% in the spleen). After the perimetamorphic period they decrease in number, although in adults aged a year or more when the thymus has involuted, a small percentage of immunoglobulin-bearing thymus cells can still be detected.

Effects of thymectomy

The increasing evidence for heterogeneity amongst lymphocytic populations in poikilotherms, and the demonstration of hapten-carrier responses in anuran, as well as in urodele amphibians (see section 5.1.4) highlight the question of the role of the thymus at this level of phylogeny.

Larval thymectomy in the midwife toad *Alytes obstetricans* reduces the response to foreign erythrocytes. Also in *X. laevis* antibody production to certain antigens is suppressed if the thymus is removed early in larval life. The thymus-dependent antigens in *X. laevis* include sheep erythrocytes (SRBC) and human gamma globulin (HGG). These same antigens are thymus-dependent in mammalian systems. However, in the absence of the

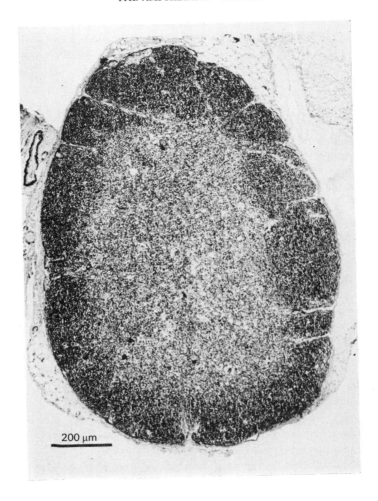

200 μm

Figure 6.7 shows a section through the thymus taken from one side of a *Xenopus laevis* toadlet. The paired single-lobed thymus of this anuran amphibian is clearly differentiated into cortex and medulla. The outer cortex is densely populated with small lymphocytes; the medulla has fewer lymphocytes, but large numbers of epithelial cells, and is less deeply stained.

From Manning, M. J. and Horton, J. D. (1974), "Functional Histogenesis of the Lymphoid Organs", pp. 263–295 in Goldspink, G. (ed.), *Differentiation and Growth of Cells in Vertebrate Tissues*, Chapman and Hall, London.

thymus in mammals, IgG to thymus-dependent antigens is completely suppressed, but IgM only partly or not at all, whereas in *X. laevis* there is an overall suppression of antibody production including all IgM. On the other hand certain antigens (e.g. bacterial lipopolysaccharide (LPS)) which are polymeric in character, have repeating antigenic determinants and are not readily degraded (see section 1.8.4), are thymus-independent in both mammals and *X. laevis*, and in both cases only IgM antibody is elicited. Thus the division into thymus-dependent and thymus-independent antibody responses extends at least as far back in phylogeny as the amphibians.

Early thymectomy in anurans has the expected effect on transplantation reactions—it results in severe deficiencies in alloimmune reactivity. In *X. laevis* the rejection of first-set grafts by thymectomized animals is a prolonged process, nevertheless it usually goes to completion. Second-set allografts from the same donor are destroyed more rapidly and within times comparable to the second-set response of control animals. It would seem that the population of lymphocytes capable of invading a graft is reduced after thymectomy, but that some capabilities remain. Possibly when the residual small population of reactive cells is expanded (either by a slow build-up of numbers in first-set responses or in second-set stimulation) graft rejection can occur. However, the source of these reactive cells is unknown, as also is the mechanism of rejection in the thymectomized animals.

The lymphoid tissues of *X. laevis* undergo relatively normal histogenesis after thymectomy. The only marked effect is on the spleen, which is reduced in size and has fewer lymphocytes in the red pulp. The absence of severe lymphoid aplasia following early thymectomy is surprising in view of the finding that in *R. pipiens* the majority of peripheral lymphocytes originate from the thymic rudiment. Perhaps there is some alternative pathway of differentiation which predominates if the thymus is destroyed, or perhaps the migration of stem cells from the thymus to the periphery is a very early ontogenetic event.

Secondary lymphoid organs

The kidney, spleen and lymph nodes of anurans are important secondary lymphoid organs and as such they show the functional characteristics of (*a*) antigen-trapping, (*b*) cellular proliferation following antigenic stimulation, and (*c*) the presence of antibody-forming cells in immunized animals.

When antigen-trapping was studied in the lymph nodes (jugular bodies) of *Bufo marinus* injected with a radioactively-labelled bacterial antigen (^{125}I-polymerized flagellin of *Salmonella adelaide*) the antigen was found by electron-microscopic autoradiography to be localized, as it is in mammalian lymph nodes, on the surface of reticular cells rather than intracellularly. Similarly, in *X. laevis* when a soluble antigen (human gamma globulin in adjuvant) was traced by immunofluorescence, its distribution in the spleen showed a pattern closely resembling that found in birds and mammals, where antigen is retained in the white pulp on the processes of dendritic cells (see figure 6.8). The fact that antigen is

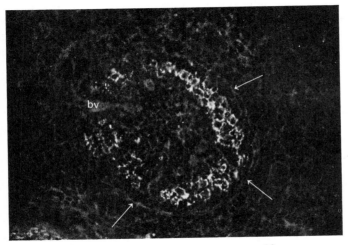

50 μm

Figure 6.8. Immunofluorescence preparation from the spleen of *Xenopus laevis* to show where antigen is localized. In this experiment the toad was injected with a soluble protein antigen (human gamma globulin). Sections of its spleen were later taken and incubated with antiserum (anti-human gamma globulin) which had been labelled with a fluorescent dye. The bright fluorescence indicates the presence of antigen which in these experiments is demonstrated within the white pulp in a peripheral zone near its border (the boundary of the white pulp is marked by arrows). The antigen is trapped in a dendritic pattern which is similar to that seen in mammals and birds where it appears to be held on surface processes of reticular cells. bv, blood vessel leaving the white pulp and emptying into the surrounding red pulp.
Courtesy of Miss Madeleine H. Collie of the University of Hull.

held on cell surfaces in a similar manner in secondary lymphoid tissues of vertebrates as dissimilar as anurans and mammals, suggests that this form of antigen-trapping is of basic importance for immune induction. Large pyroninophilic cells appear in the region where antigen is retained. These cells are involved in the proliferative response to the antigen. However, they are not organized into closely packed rounded accumulations to which the term *germinal centre* could be applied. The usual lack of germinal centres resembling those of birds and mammals has been correlated with the poor secondary responses of poikilotherms to certain antigens, since germinal centres are believed to be primary sites for immunological memory in higher vertebrates. Nevertheless, we can see from anurans that some secondary reactivity is possible even without these structures.

The presence of specific antibody-forming cells in the spleen, kidney and lymph nodes of anurans is well established. They have been demonstrated by the techniques of immunofluorescence, immunocytoadherence (rosette-forming cells and bacterial adherence) and by the detection of plaque-forming cells (PFC). *Bufo marinus* has been well studied in this respect. The antibody-forming cells to *Salmonella adelaide* antigens revealed by bacterial immunocytoadherence in kidney, spleen and lymph nodes included many lymphocytes, with a heterogeneity of cell size. Plasma cells have been detected in these organs by immunofluorescence and ultrastructural studies. They resemble mammalian plasma cells in possessing a rough vesicled endoplasmic reticulum and well-developed Golgi apparatus; in toads injected with bovine serum albumin (BSA) they appeared in greatest numbers in the kidney.

Lymphoid tissue of liver and kidney. The lymphoid tissues of the kidney and liver comprise simple accumulations of lymphocytes situated in close proximity to the blood sinuses. Cells in the liver phagocytose blood- and lymph-borne particles. Lymphocytes occur in its subcapsular area and are occasionally found in small foci associated with the phagocytosed material within the liver parenchyma.

The kidney contains lymphocytic accumulations in its intertubular tissue, often near the blood sinuses in areas where the blood flow is probably sufficiently slow to permit easy passage of lymphocytes out of the circulation to cluster in response to the presence of antigens. A lymphocytic accumulation in the kidney of *X. laevis* is shown in figure 6.9. Antigen may arrive in the kidney by several mechanisms. It may be free in the circulation; it may be carried in mobile macrophages which have taken it up elsewhere, or it may be phagocytosed by cells of the renal tubules. The latter possibility has an interesting evolutionary history dating from the primitive open nephric units (see figure 3.2) which drained fluid from the body cavity of the earliest vertebrates. It may not be entirely coincidental that in groups where functional open nephrostomes still occur, at least in larval forms, the kidney has an important role in the immune system. It is a major lymphoid organ in fishes and amphibians, but this function wanes in the kidneys of amniotes, where correspondingly greater emphasis on other secondary lymphoid organs occurs. The more highly evolved anurans, with their lymphoid kidney and rudimentary lymph nodes, possibly represent a transitional stage in these changing roles within the secondary lymphoid system.

Spleen. The lymphoid component of the spleen has a more complex architecture than that of the liver and kidney. The organ comprises a number of white pulp areas separated from the red pulp by boundary layer cells. The white pulp contains considerable numbers of small lymphocytes which surround a central arteriole as in the mammalian

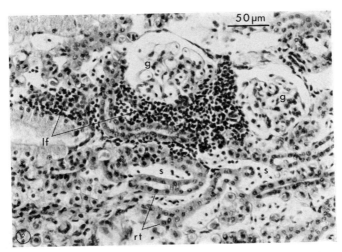

Figure 6.9. Section from the kidney of a toad (*Xenopus laevis*) showing a lymphocytic accumulation. The lymphoid focus (lf) is irregular in shape and consists of lymphocytes (with deeply stained nuclei) packed together in spaces between the renal tissue in close proximity to the renal blood sinuses (s). rt, renal tubules; g, glomerulus.

From Turner, R. J. (1973), "Response of the Toad *Xenopus laevis* to Circulating Antigens. II. Responses after Splenectomy", *Journal of Experimental Zoology*, **183**, 35–46.

spleen. A specialized antigen-trapping area occurs in the peripheral zone of the white pulp in *X. laevis*. The red pulp also contains lymphocytes, and these often form extrafollicular cuffs around the white pulp areas. It is these extrafollicular lymphocytes which are depleted after thymectomy in *X. laevis*, a finding which suggests that the territory of thymus-dependent lymphocytes may differ in amphibians and mammals, since in mammals T-cells occupy a periarteriolar region around the central arteriole. This hints at phylogenetic differences in the migratory pathways of lymphocytes, and at the same time serves to emphasize the general lack of information about lymphocytic circulation in poikilotherms (see section 4.2.5).

In *X. laevis* the spleen is the only lymphoid organ with any complexity of structural organization. These anurans lack lymph nodes and the remaining foci, such as those in the kidney, consist of irregularly arranged accumulations of lymphocytes. It is of interest, therefore, that after splenectomy good antibody production to both soluble and particulate circulating antigens can still be demonstrated. This indicates that complex structural organization of lymphoreticular tissues may not be essential to immunological competence. With threshold doses of antigen, however, the splenectomized animals failed to respond as well as intact controls. Thus the extra-splenic sites may lack the efficiency of the spleen in dealing with small amounts of antigen.

Lymph nodes. Secondary lymphoid organs similar to lymph nodes make their first appearance in evolutionary terms at the level of the amphibians, where they occur in the more advanced anurans as small nodular structures in the throat and axillary region. The lymph nodes of a leopard frog *R. pipiens* are pictured in the dissection shown in figure 6.10. The paired jugular bodies (so-called because they lie immediately ventral to the external jugular veins) are the most conspicuous lymph nodes in *Rana spp.* and *Bufo spp.* Other organs include the propericardial bodies, the procoracoid bodies and the epithelial bodies. These organs have a lymphocytic parenchyma arranged around blood sinusoids. Antigen is trapped by macrophages in the parenchyma, and by reticuloendothelial cells lining the sinusoids. The organs filter blood rather than lymph. Larval lymph glands such as that of *R. pipiens* pictured in figure 6.11, have a similar sinusoidal structure. These develop in and project into the anterior lymphatic channel, and they apparently filter lymph as well as blood.

Lymphocytes of gut and skin. Lymphoid accumulations occur in close association with the epithelium throughout much of the gastrointestinal

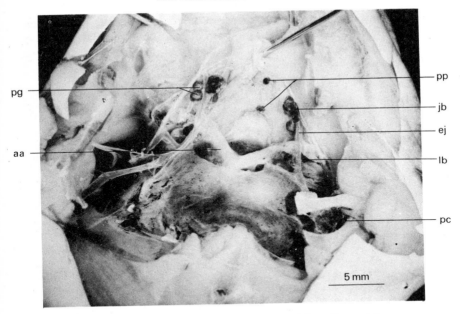

pg

aa

pp

jb

ej

lb

pc

5 mm

Figure 6.10. Ventral dissection of the leopard frog *Rana pipiens,* displaying the lymphoid organs of the throat and axillary regions. This animal had previously received an intraperitoneal injection of India ink which blackens these phagocytic organs. The paired lymphoid organs seen in this dissection include the jugular bodies (jb), the propericardial bodies (pp), the procoracoid bodies (pc) and the lympho-myeloid body (lb). aa, aortic arches; ej, external jugular vein; pg, para-thyroid glands.

From Horton, J. D. (1971), "Ontogeny of the Immune System in Amphibians", *American Zoologist,* **11,** 219–228.

tract from mouth to hind gut in both larval and adult anurans. In the larvae these include large foci, such as the ventral cavity bodies of the pharynx (see figure 6.6) and oesophageal accumulations; the exact locations vary somewhat from species to species. In the adult, more prominent nodules of gut-associated lymphoid tissue are present. These are similar in size to a single nodule of a mammalian Peyer's patch (figure 6.12) but they lack germinal centres. No structure comparable to the avian bursa of Fabricius has been detected. Lymphocytic areas are also found in the skin, e.g. in the region dorso-caudal to the fore-limb in *X. laevis.* The lymphocytes in these gut and skin accumulations occur both in the subepithelial connective tissue and within the epithelium itself. The organs show little evidence of histological change in response to antigens circulating in the blood stream, although capillaries can be seen within them; more probably they are responsive to antigenic stimulation via the gut lumen and body surface respectively.

Bone marrow. Bone marrow occurs in post-metamorphic anurans and functions as a site of haemopoiesis. Lymphoid cells are found alongside

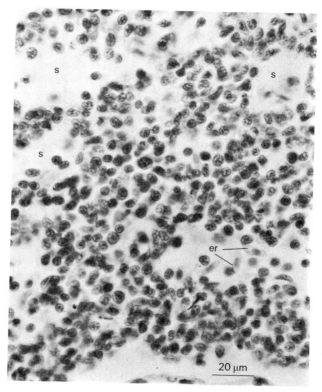

Figure 6.11.   Histology of a rudimentary lymph node of an amphibian. This section of the larval lymph gland of the leopard frog *Rana pipiens* shows blood sinuses (s) surrounded by a deeply stained parenchyma. The parenchyma contains many lymphocytes; these form simple accumulations in close proximity to the sinuses. er, erythrocyte in a blood sinus.

From Manning, M. J. and Horton, J. D. (1974), "Functional Histogenesis of the Lymphoid Organs", pp. 263–295 in Goldspink, G. (ed.). *Differentiation and Growth of Cells in Vertebrate Tissues,* Chapman and Hall, London.

the other developing blood cells in the extra-vascular fatty tissue, and they are also apparent within the capillaries of the marrow. The occurrence of bone marrow in adult anurans heralds the first regular appearance of this tissue in vertebrates.

6.1.6. *Lymphokine factors*

Information for poikilotherms on the occurrence of soluble agents of cell-mediated immunity (the lymphokine factors—see section 1.8.4, iii, and figure 1.15) is minimal. There are, however, studies which indicate the presence of a macrophage migration inhibition (MIF-like) factor in amphibians. Thus, toads *Bufo bufo* which had been immunized with tubercle mycobacteria in the form of BCG vaccine (Bacille Calmette-

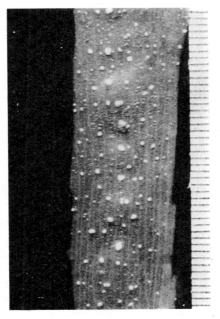

Figure 6.12. Part of the distal small intestine of the marine toad *Bufo marinus*. The gut was opened, treated with acetic acid to remove the surface epithelium, and flushed with saline. This treatment reveals a number of white elevated structures; these are simple nodules of gut-associated lymphoid tissue. Each scale division is 1 mm.
   From Goldstine, S. N., Manickavel, V. and Cohen, N. (1975), "Phylogeny of Gut-associated Lymphoid Tissue", *American Zoologist*, **15**, 107–118.

Guérin) in adjuvant and killed four weeks later, produced cells which could be harvested from their spleens and peritoneal exudates, and which when cultured in the presence of the antigen (purified protein derivative of the tubercle) plus macrophages caused an inhibition of macrophage migration. If this factor from toads is indeed a homologue of the mammalian T-cell secretion MIF, its evolutionary origin must date back to at least the early tetrapods. It is not known whether the toad factor is thymus-dependent, but studies of this kind and a search for similar factors among other poikilothermic groups would obviously be rewarding.

6.2. Conclusions

The emergence from water to land was probably the most significant step in vertebrate evolution. It involved profound modifications of the vertebrate body, and it is not surprising that these were also accompanied by changes in the immune system. Thus the kidney's role as a lymphoid organ alters with the evolution of the amniote metanephros, adaptations of the skeleton provide sites for bone marrow and, perhaps most importantly, the efficient and rapid circulation in the high-pressure blood vascular system affects migrations of immune cells from vessels to tissues. It is probably not coincidental that a diversity of immunoglobulin classes occurs at this time, since evolutionary changes in the hydrostatic and colloid osmotic pressures of the blood affect the distribution of immunoglobulins. Indeed it is possible that the various low-molecular-weight classes found in different tetrapod groups are separate innovations which arose independently in relation to movements of anti-body into the extra-vascular compartment.

The acquisition of bone marrow as a site of stem cell haemopoiesis is presumably related to the possession of the type of hollow bone structure evolved in relation to locomotion on land. Although some fish bear haemopoietic tissue in association with the cranial skeleton, fish bones are not in general suitable for this purpose. At first, bone marrow may simply represent a re-housing of stem cell populations previously situated elsewhere in the body. We do not know when it assumes importance as a B-cell stem source, but there are indications of thymus-bone marrow interactions in the leopard frog *R. pipiens*.

The anurans are the first vertebrates to possess simple lymph nodes. It is doubtful at this stage of evolution whether these represent anything more than additional organs with sinusoidal blood flow which, like the kidney, provide sites where lymphoid cells can cluster and respond to the presence of antigen. Nevertheless, the larval lymph gland develops in relation to a lymphatic channel, and this represents the type of arrangement from which the complex lymph-filtering mammalian nodes may have evolved.

CHAPTER SEVEN

THE EARLY AMNIOTES: REPTILES

7.1. Reptilia

Compared with the wealth of information available for the amphibians, reptiles have received scant attention. Alligators and boa constrictors do not, it seems, rank highly as laboratory animals, and are unlikely to lend themselves readily to immunological investigation! Nevertheless, as a group the reptiles hold an interesting phylogenetic position: (*a*) they are the closest ancestors of the birds and mammals, yet are still poikilothermic; (*b*) they are the most primitive vertebrates in which the young develop within a protected environment created by the amnion. This latter characteristic means that reptiles lack some of the experimental advantages that the free-living amphibians can offer, but at the same time it means that there is no longer a pressing need for an immune system during the early stages of the individual's development, which in turn may present a new opportunity at this phylogenetic level for refinements to be made to the immune system before bringing it into play.

The existing reptiles represent only four of the dozen or more main lines that have been identified in the fossil record. The Chelonia (tortoises and turtles) retain some of the characteristics of the earliest Permian reptiles; the Rhynchocephalia, represented by the rare protected New Zealand tuatara *Sphenodon punctatum*, survive with little change from the Triassic period; The successful Squamata (lizards and snakes) are a modern group descended from forms related to the tuatara; and the Crocodilia, though an aberrant group, are related to the bird stock (see figure 7.1).

7.1.1. *Transplantation reactions*

The speed of skin graft rejection in reptiles is temperature-dependent as in other poikilotherms. However, even at moderate temperatures (mid-20s), chronic rejection of first-set skin allografts is the rule: Chelonia, Squamata and Crocodilia all show slow rejection times (Table 7.1). Specific memory can be demonstrated by second- and third-set grafting, where rejection is accelerated. Experiments using lizards, *Calotes versicolor.* injected with anti-*Calotes* thymocyte (thymus lymphocyte) serum raised in rabbits have shown that skin graft survival times are prolonged in these animals, suggesting that reptilian cells of thymic origin are involved in the graft rejection process.

7.1.2. *Graft-versus-host reactions*

Spleen cells from one snapping turtle *Chelydra serpentina*, injected intra-peritoneally into newly hatched animals of the same species, may lead to death of the recipient: the immunocompetent donor cells react against the host, while the latter's immunological defences are unable to kill the injected cells (figure 7.2). It can be seen from Table 7.2 that, if graft and host come from remote geographical regions (where there has been no chance of interbreeding), there is a higher mortality rate in the hosts than when they originate from the same locality as the donor (and are likely to be more closely related to it). Host spleen enlargement (splenomegaly) is

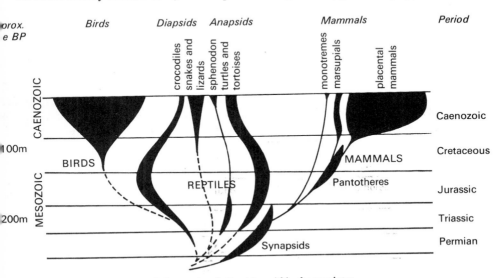

Figure 7.1.   Phylogenetic relationships within the amniotes
The distribution through time of the different groups of amniotes (reptiles, birds and mammals) is shown. BP, time before the present in millions of years.

Table 7.1. Skin allograft rejection in reptiles*

Animal	Temperature (°C)	MST† (and/or range) First-set	Second-set (days)
Chelydra serpentina (snapping turtle)	25	47(41–70)	25(20–32)
Anolis carolinensis (chamaeleon)	23·5	60–90	—
Cnemidophorus sexlineatus (race runner lizard)	—	more than 26	—
Ctenosaura pectinata (iguana)	25	48–87	30–86
Calotes versicolor (bloodsucker lizard)	29–33	45 (approx.)	—
Xantusia vigilis (yucca night lizard)	20	21–245	—
Thamnophis sirtalis (garter snake)	25	41(31–53)	25(21–29)
Caiman sclerops (caiman)	25–27	more than 65 (25—more than 110)	—

* From Borysenko, M. (1970), "Transplantation Immunity in Reptilia," *Transplantation Proceedings*, **11**, 299–306 (with modifications).

† MST: mean or median survival time.

also more evident in the first group, and death usually occurs more rapidly. The severity of the reptilian graft-versus-host reaction thus appears to be associated with the degree of genetic disparity between the graft and the host. Table 7.2 also shows that there is a greater mortality in both groups of recipients at 30 °C than at 20 °C. The chronic nature of the skin graft reaction in snapping turtles (Table 7.1) suggests an absence of strong histocompatibility antigens in this animal; the increased

Table 7.2. Graft-versus-host reactions in snapping turtles*

Geographical origin donor	host	Temperature	Mortality of hosts†
Wisconsin	New York	30 °C	19/26 (73%)
Wisconsin	Wisconsin	30 °C	10/21 (48%)
Wisconsin	New York	20 °C	8/23 (35%)
Wisconsin	Wisconsin	20 °C	4/21 (19%)

* From: Borysenko, M. and Tulipan, P. (1973), "The Graft-versus-host Reaction in the Snapping Turtle *Chelydra serpentina*," *Transplantation*, **16**, 496–504 (with modifications).

† Number of animals dead within 120 days/total number (%) after injection of 5×10^6 allogeneic spleen cells per animal: all cells were derived from a single adult Wisconsin donor.

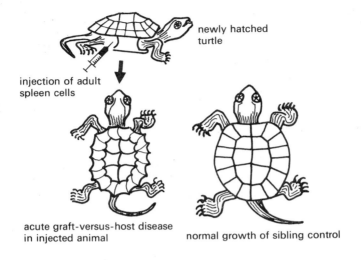

newly hatched
turtle

injection of adult
spleen cells

acute graft-versus-host disease
in injected animal

normal growth of sibling control

Figure 7.2.   Graft-versus-host reaction in a turtle
Part of the experiment shown in Table 7.2, in which newly hatched
turtles were injected intraperitoneally with adult spleen cells is
illustrated. This treatment can lead to graft-versus-host reactivity,
which results in weight loss, softening of the shell, increase in spleen
size, and in many cases rapid death.

intensity of graft-versus-host reactions found in genetically disparate
pairings and at higher temperatures may therefore be due to the additive
effects of many weak histocompatibility antigens.

7.1.3. *Antibody production*

The capacity of reptiles to produce antibody to soluble and particulate
antigens is temperature-dependent, with generally prolonged responses
yielding antibodies of low titre. Intraspecific antibodies (allohaemag-
glutinins) have been detected in a number of reptilian species; where
intraspecific haemagglutinins are not detectable, interspecific haemagglutinins can be. The predominant immunoglobulin is a high-molecular-
weight (18–19S) macroglobulin of the IgM type. Although there has been
no detailed account of the existence of IgG molecules (with a γ-type heavy
chain) in reptiles, immunoglobulin classes other than IgM do exist: turtles,
for example, possess a low-molecular-weight immunoglobulin with heavy

chains similar to those of the class termed IgN, found in the lungfish (see section 4.2.4) and other vertebrates; and tuatara serum contains a 7S globulin, the heavy chains of which are antigenically different from the μ-chains of its high-molecular-weight (IgM) immunoglobulin.

The type of immunoglobulin produced in response to antigenic challenge depends in part on the nature of the antigen injected. In lizards, *Tiliqua rugosa*, immunized with rat erythrocytes or bovine serum albumin, a high-molecular-weight (19S) mercaptoethanol-sensitive antibody appears first and persists for a long time, but a 7S mercaptoethanol-resistant antibody does appear late in the response; the same species produces only high-molecular-weight (19S) antibody against *Salmonella typhimurium*, even as late as 240 days post-immunization. Similarly in the tuatara *Sphenodon punctatum*, the anti-*Salmonella adelaide* antibody is confined to the high-molecular-weight (18S) immunoglobulin type even after 252 days (in contrast to the mammalian response to the same antigen, where a shift from 19S to 7S is soon observed). The tortoise *Testudo ibera* showed only high-molecular-weight antibody to *Brucella abortus* but, in another tortoise (the European pond tortoise *Emys orbicularis*), a soluble protein antigen, bovine serum albumin, elicited production of high-molecular-weight (19S) antibody, followed eventually by a low-molecular-weight (7S) component. The demonstration of only high-molecular-weight (IgM) antibody in response to the bacterial antigens in these reptilian experiments is reminiscent of findings in amphibians. The differing antibody response to different types of antigen probably reflects differences in the way the antigens are processed on entering the body. The number of antigen injections the animal has received can also influence the type of antibody elicited: on primary immunization with pig serum, tortoises *Testudo hermanii* first produce high molecular weight (18S) then 7S antibodies, both of which are 2-mercaptoethanol-sensitive; on secondary stimulation these are joined by a 2-mercaptoethanol-resistant 7S antibody, the amount of which increases with each additional immunization; finally a fourth antibody type (4·5S) may be demonstrated after the fourth immunization.

Secondary antibody responses

Several reptiles appear capable of secondary antibody responses, but the form this memory takes is variable. Tortoises, besides showing qualitative immunoglobulin changes due to repeated stimulation with pig serum that we have just described, respond to sheep erythrocytes more rapidly on a second stimulation, although no increase in antibody titres is seen. Similarly, secondary stimulation of lizards, *Calotes versicolor*, with sheep cells elicits a more rapid rise in the numbers of antibody-forming cells and serum antibody levels with a shorter latent period than in a primary response, but again there is no increase in the amount of antibody produced. On the other hand, the desert iguana *Dipsosaurus dorsalis* shows a 3–4 fold increase in titre after secondary stimulation with keyhole limpet haemocyanin, and the lizard *Tiliqua rugosa* has been shown to produce higher titres of antibody following a secondary stimulation with rat erythrocytes or with *Salmonella typhimurium*. It is worth recalling here that the rat cells elicit both 19S and 7S antibodies, the *Salmonella* just 19S, suggesting that secondary responsiveness in reptiles need not necessarily be associated with a change in the type of antibody produced, although in *Sphenodon punctatum* immunized with *Salmonella adelaide*, which also elicits only macroglobulin, no secondary antibody response could be demonstrated.

7.1.4. *Ontogeny of the immune system*

In the snapping turtle there is good evidence of a late maturation of the immune system. Firstly, the graft-versus-host phenomenon discussed in section 7.1.2 shows a deficiency in the allogeneic reactivity of newly-hatched turtles, since they succumb to injected spleen cells from an unrelated adult; secondly, spleen explants from adult but not young turtles can form haemagglutinating antibodies against xenogeneic erythrocytes; thirdly, the ability to reject skin xenografts and allografts matures only 4–6 months after hatching. It is tempting to correlate this slow maturation of the turtle immune system (compared with that of anuran amphibians, for example) with the amniote condition. However, generalizations on the strength of this one "representative" species are somewhat dangerous at present, since lizards (*Calotes*) have shown different results. Here the ability to produce antibodies against xenogeneic erythrocytes is already developed at the time of hatching, and the number of antibody-forming cells expressed as a percentage of the total cells is higher than in adults. Moreover, adult lizard spleen cells injected into newly hatched lizards do not bring about a graft-versus-host reaction, thus demonstrating an earlier ability in this reptile to respond to alloantigens also. Further studies are needed in this area.

7.1.5. *Lymphoid tissues*

Lymphoid tissues in reptiles include the bone marrow, thymus and spleen, all of which have their equivalents in other, higher and lower, vertebrate classes. During development, there is a very long vitelline haemopoiesis in these primitive amniotes, which lasts up to 18 days after fertilization. Then the bone marrow and liver begin to produce lymphocytes. In some reptiles at least (e.g. *Chelydra*), the bone marrow can become the source of all kinds of lymphoid cells.

The thymus

The reptilian thymus develops from the dorsal pharyngeal epithelium as in nearly all other vertebrates (figure 7.3), and the differentiated organ

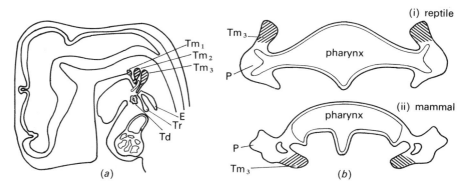

Figure 7.3. Embryological development of the thymus

(a) Vertical section of an embryonic lizard *Lacerta agilis* showing dorsal thymic outgrowths from the first three pharyngeal pouches. The thymic buds from the first pair of pharyngeal pouches (Tm_1) are transitory. The buds from the second and third pairs (Tm_2 and Tm_3) give rise to the definitive adult thymus in the lizard. E, oesophagus; Td, thyroid; Tr, trachea.

(b) Transverse sections through the region of the third pair of pharyngeal pouches in (i) a reptile and (ii) a mammal: a diagrammatic representation comparing the origin of the thymus in these two vertebrate classes. In the reptiles, as in most other vertebrates, the thymus arises from the dorsal part of the pouch; in the mammals it is more ventral in origin. Tm_3, thymic bud; P, region of development of the parathyroid.

After Maurer 1899; diagram (a) redrawn after Bockman, D. E. (1970), "The Thymus", in *Biology of the Reptilia*, Gans, C. and Parsons, T. S., eds. **3**, 111–133, Academic Press, London and New York.

is histologically comparable to that in other groups. Different pairs of pharyngeal pouches yield the thymic buds in different groups of reptiles: in lizards the thymus develops from the 2nd and 3rd, in snakes from the 4th and 5th and in turtles from the 3rd and 4th pharyngeal pouches. The adult thymus in turtles is found near the angle formed by the division of the subclavian and common carotid arteries, in snakes it is situated anterior to the heart, while in crocodiles it extends forward from a broad posterior portion near the heart into the cervical region where it lies along almost the entire length of the neck; this bird-like location of the crocodile's thymus is interesting in view of the phylogenetic relationship between the Aves and the Crocodilia.

Age involution of the reptilian thymus has been reported and the organ also shows seasonal fluctuations in weight, the latter being a transitory variation (low in winter, high in summer) superimposed upon the overall decrease in size due to age changes. Seasonal involution of the thymus is a common occurrence in vertebrates: it is also seen, for example, in amphibians (e.g. *Rana esculenta*) and in birds (see section 8.1.7). The role of the reptilian thymus has been little studied; apart from recent experiments which implicate the thymus in skin graft rejection (see section 7.1.1), few functional comparisons with other vertebrate classes can yet be made.

The spleen, liver and kidney

In the lizard *Lacerta*, the spleen differentiates at 27 days post-fertilization, which is late compared with anuran amphibians. The differentiated spleen in a number of diverse reptiles—the tuatara (*Sphenodon*), lizards (*Tiliqua* and *Calotes*) and turtles (*Chelydra*), for example—reveals a more or less clear separation into white pulp and red pulp, a feature which is common to most vertebrate spleens from fish to mammals. However, germinal centres, clearly defined in the spleen and other lymphoid tissues of birds and mammals, are absent. The spleen in reptiles appears to play a more dominant role in antibody production than it does in lower vertebrates such as fish and amphibia. Splenectomized lizards (*Calotes*) are completely unable to produce antibodies against sheep erythrocytes; attempts to locate the antibody-forming cells in intact specimens of *Calotes* and in the tortoise *Testudo* have found them only in the spleen and blood, although in the desert iguana (*Dipsosaurus*) some antibody-forming cells were detected in the liver also. In the lizard *Tiliqua*, a few lymphocytes have been found in the portal tracts of the liver, but they lack any organized morphology. The kidney of this reptile also contains small simple pockets of lymphoid cells, some of which may synthesize antibody to rat erythro-cytes, but it is not known whether they were stimulated in the kidney or migrated there.

Electron-microscope studies of cells shown by direct methods to be antibody-forming cells in tortoise (*Agrionemys*) spleens have revealed con-siderable variations in the cell type involved. Some antibody-forming cells were morphologically unspecialized, with a spherical nucleus, slightly developed endoplasmic reticulum and numerous ribosomes, most of which were not adhering to the endoplasmic reticulum. Mostly, however, the cells possessed an irregular eccentric nucleus, and a moderate amount of endoplasmic reticulum with sac-like cisterni. None of the antibody-forming cells in these experiments possessed the characteristically layered endoplasmic reticulum of the mammalian plasma cell. Earlier studies have reported plasma cells in spleens of turtles and alligators, especially following repeated antigenic stimulation, and in the lungs of garter snakes, but these studies relied entirely on morphological criteria: it has not been established that the cells observed were actually involved in antibody production.

Gut-associated lymphoid tissue

In view of the affinities between reptiles and birds, several workers have looked for reptilian equivalents of the avian bursa of Fabricius, an organ found in the cloacal region which plays such an important part (as the source of B-lymphocytes) in the establishment of the avian immune system. In snapping turtles, about 20 lymphoid aggregations have regularly been found projecting into the cloacal lumen, lying directly below the mucosa; similar aggregations are present in tortoises (*Testudo*) and snakes (*Elaphe*), but are less prominent in alligators. Unlike the avian bursa which, together with the thymus, assumes its major function early in development, the cloacal lymphocytes in the turtles were less in evidence in the newly hatched animal than in the adult. It has been reported that other turtles (*Chrysemys*) and *Sphenodon* lack any sign of a bursa equivalent.

Reptilian lymphoid tissues have also been observed in various locations in more anterior regions of the gut. The oesophagus and small intestine of the snake (*Elaphe*), for example, possess discrete nodules in the mucosa plus more diffuse lymphoid tissue, whilst the latter type only is seen in the stomach and large intestine. As in the snake, snapping turtles show lymphoid foci in the small intestine, which might be related to Peyer's patches in mammals. Tonsil-like organs are also found in these turtles and in alligators.

Primitive lymph nodes

"True" lymph nodes of the mammalian type connected into afferent and efferent lymphatics, are not found in reptiles. However, a somewhat motley collection of nodes which may be related to the mammalian structures and/or to the lymphoid aggregates seen scattered along lymphatic trunks in birds, has been described. In lymph sinuses surrounding the aorta, vena cava and internal jugular veins of the snake *Elaphe*, for example, nodules are seen which protrude into the lumen from the wall. Similar nodules, related to the lymphatic system, occur in the gekko *Gehyra variegata* where lymphoid tissue investing the lateral vein is associated with the perivascular axillary lymph sinus. Nodes have also been described in the lizard *Tiliqua*, close to the ventral surface of the body, adjacent to the foreleg; while in turtles (*Chelydra*), lymphoid organs have been seen in the inguinal and axillary regions of the body, corresponding in location to certain mammalian lymph nodes, although they apparently filter blood rather than lymph. *Sphenodon* and *Alligator*, on the other hand, are reported to be devoid of lymph nodes of any description.

7.2. Conclusions

Compared with many amphibians, some reptiles show a delayed onset of immunocompetence and slow differentiation of lymphoid organs which may be related to their amniote status, although more studies are needed to verify this. On the other hand, there is as yet little indication that the levels of immunocompetence finally attained in reptiles are significantly more sophisitcated than in other poikilothermic vertebrates; skin graft rejection is slow, and antibody production not particularly vigorous. Selection pressures governing the production of high versus low-molecular-weight antibodies appear to be quite different in reptiles and other poikilothermic vertebrates from those in mammals. Both can replace their high-molecular-weight IgM with low-molecular-weight immunoglobulins during the course of immunization to many antigens, but mammals do so rapidly and as a matter of course, whereas reptiles do not: IgM is predominant. These differences are likely to be due in part to differences in body temperature, but they may also reflect differences in the efficiency of their immunological effector mechanisms. Lymphoid organization is simpler in all groups of reptiles than in birds and mammals, even though the beginnings of more specialized structures such as Peyer's patches and lymph nodes may exist in some species.

CHAPTER EIGHT

HOMOIOTHERMIC VERTEBRATES: BIRDS

8.1. Aves

Although birds are placed in a separate class of vertebrates (Aves), they are closely related to the reptiles and show obvious affinities with the diapsid stock which includes all modern reptiles except the chelonians; their closest living relatives are the Crocodilia. Phylogenetically the birds are clearly separated from the mammals but share with them a homoiothermic status with all the improved physiological efficiency, mastery of diverse environmental conditions and high metabolic demands which this entails. The modifications of the internal environment which accompany homoiothermy affect invading organisms as well as host tissues, and may well provide an evolutionary incentive for the vigorous and prompt immune responses displayed by both of these vertebrate groups. Indeed in many aspects of their physiology the birds rival—and sometimes surpass—the mammals; this is true of their cellular and humoral immune capabilities.

Much of the research on birds has been done with the domestic chicken—no doubt because of the expertise available for rearing and handling these birds, and because of their importance to the poultry industry. A major incentive for work on birds has been the clear delineation of T-cell and B-cell systems in this group, with the resulting widespread use of the bursectomized chicken as a model of the B-cell deficient state (see section 8.1.7). A further boost has come with the recent availability of suitable inbred lines.

8.1.1. Transplantation reactions

Birds show acute rejection of allografted tissue with rapid first-set responses and clear-cut second-set memory. Chicks become fully competent in their alloimmune responses a few days after hatching. Acute rejection in the chicken is controlled by a major histocompatibility

127

system—the B system. This chromosomal region simultaneously functions as a major histocompatibility locus and as a blood-group locus. As a blood-group system, B shows extensive polymorphism with at least 21 alleles. Skin grafts exchanged between birds which are incompatible at the B-locus show an onset of rejection at about 7 days in the first-set response and at 3 to 4 days in second-set responses. In contrast, chickens compatible at the B-locus but differing at weaker loci, may show chronic rejection times of 40 days or more. Minor histocompatibilities in the chicken include a sex-linked histocompatibility antigen. Since the female is the heterogametic sex in birds, it is the graft "female to male" (ZW to ZZ) which is rejected, the opposite of the "male to female" (XY to XX) sex-linked histoincompatibility in mice.

During normal skin-graft rejection in birds, there is a lymphocytic infiltration of the graft bed which is accompanied by the appearance of plasma cells and liberation into the serum of specific cytotoxic antibodies. These cytotoxic antibodies are not essential for graft rejection: bursectomized birds do not produce them, but are still fully competent in their transplantation reactions—at least to tissue grafts, although there is some evidence that their response to cells administered in suspension is impaired. Similarly, skin allografts surviving on specifically tolerant chickens are destroyed if the tolerant animals are given sensitized lymphoid cells, but not after administration of immune serum (i.e. they are rejected by a cell-mediated mechanism). On the other hand, in inbred ducks, transfer of transplantation immunity by means of specific IgG alloantibodies has been reported, although this reaction is complex and lymphocytes are still essential.

8.1.2. Graft-versus-host reactions

The chorio-allantoic membrane of the hen's egg is a highly suitable site for the growth of organisms and tissues, and has long been used for this purpose. This led to one of the earlier demonstrations of graft-versus-host reactivity. Thus if the cells which are transplanted come from the same species as the egg, and are immunologically competent, they will set up an alloimmune reaction against the embryo, which is itself too immature to reject them. The reaction is measured by the occurrence of lesions (pocks) on the chorio-allantoic membrane and by enlargement of the host's spleen. This provides a convenient test for the presence of immunocompetent donor cells and permits quantitation; e.g. by inoculating a known number of cells on to the chorio-allantoic membrane and counting the pocks which they produce (see figure 8.1). In experiments where splenic enlargement is used as the criterion of graft-versus-host reactivity, the cells are usually injected intravenously.

It has been shown that graft-versus-host reactions occur when there is a major histocompatibility difference between donor and host; indeed, the presence of large pocks on the chorio-allantoic membrane on the 4th day after inoculation is indicative of a major histoincompatibility associated

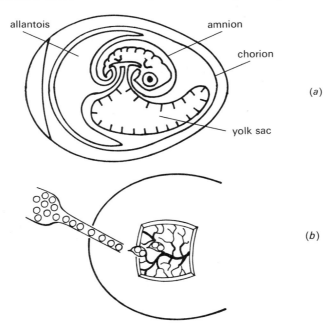

allantois

amnion

chorion

(a)

yolk sac

(b)

Figure 8.1.   Use of chorio-allantoic membrane for grafting experiments

(a) Diagram (a) shows the extra-embryonic membranes of the chick. After Balinsky, B. I. (1960), *An Introduction to Embryology*, W. B. Saunders Company, Philadelphia and London.

(b) Transplantation on to the chorio-allantoic membrane. The chorio-allantoic membrane lies immediately below the shell membrane. Its vessels can be seen by "candling" the egg. An area with good vascularization is selected, the shell carefully removed above the area, and the shell membrane moistened and peeled away to expose the chorio-allantoic membrane. The graft of tissues or cells is then placed on the chorio-allantoic membrane near a blood vessel as shown in diagram (b). The shell is put back, and the egg incubated for a further period and then examined, e.g. in the graft-versus-host reaction for the presence of pocks on the chorio-allantoic membrane and/or enlargement of the spleen.

with the B-locus. Furthermore, the intensity of the graft-versus-host reaction is controlled by this locus. Thus lines of White Leghorn chickens homozygous for the allele B^{14} are excellent graft-versus-host donors, while lines homozygous for B^2 give poor responses as donors, and the heterozygote B^{12}/B^2 shows intermediate capabilities. The reaction is one between lymphoid cells of the donor and haemopoietic cells of the host. If the host is a young embryo, the elements of its yolk sac blood islands are inactivated. In older embryos, the derivatives of cells from these blood islands are stimulated to divide (on the chorio-allantoic membrane, in the spleen and elsewhere), and the proliferative events in the graft-versus-host reaction in fact involve both donor and host cells. Blood cells from a late embryo at the 20th day of incubation are already capable of causing graft-versus-host reactions if inoculated as donor cells into another embryo; this is a good demonstration of their immunocompetence. The host chick itself becomes able to resist the induction of graft-versus-host reactivity a few days after hatching.

8.1.3. *The major histocompatibility system*

The availability of inbred lines of chickens has given impetus to studies of their major histocompatibility system. It is now known that the mixed lymphocyte reaction in birds is controlled by a gene or genes mapping to the B-gene region. Thus lymphoid cells from the blood of chickens which have the same major histocompatibility antigens (B-antigens) give consistently negative results when tested for mixed lymphocyte reactivity, while lines which differ at the B-locus always show positive stimulation. The B-locus is also involved in the regulation of delayed hypersensitivity reactions to tuberculin, and it has been implicated in overall fitness and disease susceptibility. Furthermore, it has recently been shown that a major gene controlling the intensity of antibody formation to the synthetic polypeptide which is generally known as (T, G)—A——L maps with the B-region in the chicken. Thus not only mammals but also birds show linkage of an antigen-specific immune response gene with the major histocompatibility locus. The most likely explanation of the similarity of the B-system of chickens to the H-2 major histocompatibility system of mice and the HL-A system of man (see section 1.3.2) is that the mammalian and avian systems have a common evolutionary origin. Such evidence as is available for reptiles tends to argue otherwise, since reptiles seem to lack major histocompatibility antigens. However, as we have seen in Chapter 7, the reptiles as a group obviously warrant more intensive investigation.

8.1.4. *Tolerance induction*

Tolerance to allogeneic cells

Parabiosis can be achieved easily in birds by joining the blood circulations of the extra-embryonic membranes. This can be done at 6–11 days of incubation by cutting a small hole in the shell overlying the most vascular region of the chorio-allantoic membrane, and aligning the membranes of the two eggs by a method which permits vascular anastomosis to develop between the chorio-allantoic blood vessels of the partners. It can also be done even earlier, at 4–5 days of incubation, by forming contacts between the chorion, area vasculosa and yolk sac region of the two embryos. The results are similar to those obtained after parabiosis in other vertebrates, i.e. mutual tolerance ensues. Indeed, one of the early demonstrations that the natural chimaerism described by Owen in free-martin cattle (see section 1.6.1) could be artificially produced in an experimental animal, was made in this way in the chicken. Thus chickens which hatched from parabiont eggs in which they had a shared blood circulation failed to make antibody to each other's erythrocytes, and retained their partner's skin when this was grafted at two weeks post-hatching. These results can also be obtained by injecting blood cells into the embryonic circulation. Furthermore, a situation occurs which is similar to that already described in amphibians (section 6.1.2): large doses of allogeneic cells induce tolerance, small doses elicit immunity. Small doses of allogeneic blood cells can sensitize an embryo from at least the age of 13 days. If the embryo is injected at this age and then tested later when it is a 2-day-old hatchling, the animal will give a second-set response to skin from the same donor; i.e. the early exposure to a small number of cells induces positive immunity and not tolerance. When larger numbers of cells are used, and tolerance is produced in the embryo, this may lead to graft-versus-host reactions as described in section 8.1.2.

Tolerance can be demonstrated not only by means of allogeneic skin grafts but also by failure of the tolerant bird to provide immunocompetent cells which can effect specific graft-versus-host reactions when used as donor cells. Bursectomized birds (see section 8.1.7) which do not produce antibody can still be rendered tolerant, a finding which eliminates the possibility that blocking factors involving circulating immunoglobulins could be responsible. Tolerance in these circumstances may be due to the modification or elimination of specifically reactive clones of cells, but there is also evidence from the chicken which suggests that there is active suppression. Thus peripheral blood cells from tolerant chickens are able to inhibit the graft-versus-host reactivity which would normally be expressed by cells taken from non-tolerant birds, i.e. active suppressor cells may be implicated.

Tolerance to soluble and particulate antigens

Tolerance can be induced to soluble antigens, such as foreign serum proteins, by injecting large doses intraperitoneally shortly after hatching. As in similar experiments with other systems, the more closely the foreign antigen resembles the animal's own proteins, the more likely it is to be tolerated. For example, turkey serum is more tolerogenic than mammalian serum in chickens, although it is less tolerogenic in a mammal.

Particulate antigens, such as foreign erythrocytes or killed *Salmonella pullorum* organisms, can also induce tolerance if presented in large doses at a sufficiently early age. Birds treated with particulate antigens have been used in experiments on the role of persisting antigen. Turkey erythrocytes, labelled with radioactive chromium and injected into newly hatched chickens, induced a state of tolerance which could be maintained, provided that additional injections of turkey erythrocytes were given whenever the level of the circulating antigen, measured by its radioactivity, fell much below the original dose. Birds kept for long intervals with only low levels of antigen were likely to lose tolerance, and this likelihood was greater for young birds than for older ones. This is similar to findings for soluble proteins in mammals, and is explained by the notion that an influx of newly produced cells is responsible for escape from tolerance. More antigen is required to render the newly formed cells tolerant when the cell turnover is high in juvenile birds than when the rate of new cell production slows down. Indeed, the number of incoming reactive cells which could respond positively to the lowered (immunogenic) levels of antigen in the older birds may be quite small.

8.1.5. *Humoral immunity in birds*

Antibody production

Birds produce both high and low-molecular-weight antibodies to a large array of antigens, and their immune processes are in general comparable with those of mammals. They even resemble mammals by occasionally making antibodies against their own tissues—an abnormal situation which gives rise to autoimmune diseases. Thus certain chicken strains show a spontaneous autoimmune disease of the thyroid which involves the formation of humoral factors and which can be prevented if antibody is suppressed by removal of the bursa of Fabricius.

Humoral immune responses in birds do, however, have certain distinctive features. The typical time course of the normal avian primary response differs from that of a mammal in its surprisingly short latent period, rapid rise to a peak, and short duration. For example, a single intravenous injection of human serum albumin into a chicken elicits a strong primary response in which circulating antibody is detectable at day 4, reaches a peak at day 8–12, and then rapidly falls to a low level by day 18. Indeed the speed of the early events in the avian reaction is more reminiscent of the secondary response of a mammal than of primary antibody production. If an adjuvant is used and injected together with the antigen at an intramuscular site, a single injection produces a first peak followed after about 3 weeks by a second peak which reaches high levels during the second month after immunization. Antibody production during this second peak occurs mainly in the inflammatory (granulomatous) tissues at the site of the injection.

In birds, as in other vertebrates, bacterial lipopolysaccharides elicit IgM antibody; the chicken responds to these antigens with a series of cyclical fluctuations in IgM production. For many other antigens, initial IgM synthesis is followed by the production of increasing amounts of low-molecular-weight antibody. The low-molecular-weight antibody to soluble antigens gives peculiar precipitation reactions in birds in that optimal precipitation of antigen-antibody complexes *in vitro* occurs at high salt concentration. Indeed, increases up to an optimum concentration of 8% sodium chloride (i.e. almost ten times the normal physiological value) result in increases both in the amount of the precipitate and the rate of the reaction. This contrasts with mammalian precipitating antibody which acts less well at high salt concentrations.

Immunoglobulin classes

The high and low-molecular-weight immunoglobulins of the chicken resemble the IgM and IgG classes of mammals in their general structural properties, although chicken "IgG" is sufficiently unlike that of the mammal to be designated "IgY" by some authors. The pentameric nature of the chicken IgM has been verified by electron microscopy. Ducks have three major immunoglobulins based on size: the IgM and two low-molecular-weight proteins sedimenting at 7·8S and at 5·7S. The 7·8S immunoglobulin of ducks is structurally similar to the chicken IgG-type, and it shows partial identity with the chicken low-molecular-weight class in immunodiffusion tests. The two duck low-molecular-weight immuno-globulins are antigenically related, and they probably belong to the same immunoglobulin class. Thus heavy chains from the 7·8S protein have antigenic determinants in common with the heavy chains from the 5·7S, although with some additional unique determinants. The 5·7S is not a local break-down product or precursor of the 7·8S molecule as evidenced by the lack of interconversion following injection of radiolabelled 5·7S or 7·8S immunoglobulins into ducks. The presence of a low-molecular-weight immune protein with relatively short heavy chain occurs not only in ducks (5·7S immunoglobulin) but also in the Dipnoi (5·9S, IgN) immuno-globulin, possibly in teleost grouper fish, and in turtles, geese, marsupials and rabbits—a puzzling array which should not at this stage be taken to imply homology since more information on primary structure and the antigenic relationships of these molecules is required before any phylo-genetic inferences can be made. In the duck almost equal amounts of 7·8S and 5·7S antibody are present early in the immune response, but in hyperimmunized animals as much as 75% of the total may be 5·7S. Both kappa and lambda type of light chain can be identified in birds; in the chicken the kappa type of light chain predominates.

Several groups of workers have identified a class of immunoglobulin in the chicken with an electrophoretic mobility similar to that of human IgA. These immunoglobulins form only a minor component of the immunoglobulins in the serum, but they are the major class in external secretions (e.g. bile, intestinal secretions, saliva, tracheal and bronchial washings, oviducts and egg white). The serum IgA of the chicken differs from chicken IgM and IgG both antigenically and in its well-marked ability to bind radio-labelled human secretory component—although a similar secretory piece has not been conclusively demonstrated in the chicken itself, which may perhaps have a different secretory component. Immunofluorescent techniques reveal the presence of avian IgA in cells of the intestinal mucosa.

There are many indications not only that birds possess a secretory immune system but also that this operates in local infections. This is borne out by experience with immunization procedures: in Newcastle disease, for example, good immunity to respiratory infection can be obtained by local immunization of the respiratory tract. However, analogy in function may not necessarily mean homology in structure. Only primary criteria from amino-acid sequences or immunological cross reactivity will establish this. To date IgA has been identified with certainty only in mammals. It now looks as though birds may have a similar system, the phylogenetic origins of which are still obscure—for, although a few preliminary studies have been made in poikilotherms, there is as yet no concrete evidence for the presence of IgA in lower vertebrates.

Immediate hypersensitivity reactions

Immediate hypersensitivity reactions have been described in chickens and in pigeons following immunization with soluble foreign proteins. The reaction can be fatal in adults, but is usually less severe in young birds. Thus, if the bird is injected as a 15-day old embryo and again with the same antigen at 3–4 days post-hatching, it may respond to the challenging dose with muscular contraction, vasodilation, defaecation and respiratory distress lasting for up to 15 minutes. Immediate hypersensitivity can be passively transferred from the sensitized bird to a recipient by the transfer of immune serum. The serum evokes a skin reaction if the recipient is subsequently challenged with antigen (passive cutaneous anaphylaxis) especially in younger birds which are more responsive owing to their greater histamine sensitivity. The reaction can be blocked by antihistamines and is probably mediated by degranulation of mast cells which release histamine and other pharmacologically active agents. This is very similar to the IgE-mediated immediate-hypersensitivity responses of mammals, but the antibody involved differs from IgE in that it is not particularly labile to heating and is 2-mercaptoethanol-resistant. Unlike IgE it remains fixed to tissue receptors for less than 72 hours rather than for an extended period of time. It more nearly resembles antibodies of an IgG subclass (IgG_1) of the guinea pig and some other mammals. Indeed, the antibody concerned in the chicken appears to be related to the IgG class. It is indistinguishable from chicken IgG antigenically, but it is biologically separable, since unlike most of the IgG it does not appear in the yolk, and it probably represents a distinct IgG subclass.

8.1.6. *Ontogeny of immunity*

Transfer of maternal antibodies

In amniotes the developing young in the uterus or in the egg are protected from much of the antigenic challenge which they will encounter after birth or hatching. Around this period antibodies synthesized by the mother and transferred to the young help to give temporary protection while the immature animal's own immune defences are getting under way. In birds, immunoglobulin is passed via the follicular epithelium in the hen's ovary into the egg yolk. This is a selective process whereby the concentration of immunoglobulin in the egg reaches many times the concentration of other serum components and in which IgG is passed preferentially. IgM and IgA which are present in the oviduct secretions are acquired with the albumin as the egg passes down the oviduct.

The developing embryo absorbs antibody from the yolk by way of the vitelline and hepatic circulations, and IgG can be detected in its serum; it appears that only IgG antibodies pass across the yolk-sac wall during embryonic life. In the chicken, as in the rabbit, selective transport has been demonstrated experimentally in that the yolk sac transmits xeno-geneic immunoglobulin less readily than immunoglobulins obtained from the animal's own species. Maternal IgA and IgM which are present in the albumin appear in the amniotic fluid. They enter the embryonic gut during the later part of the incubation period, when swallowing movements of the embryo result in intake of the amniotic fluid with which the albumin is mixed. Thus in birds, as in mammals, there may be a different mode of transmission for maternal immunoglobulins of different classes. In many mammals passive transfer of maternal antibody after birth occurs in the mammary secretions, but in birds it must all be present in the egg. However, the newly-hatched chick, unlike the newborn mammal, still retains the yolk sac which is retracted into the abdomen, thus some passively acquired antibody is still available after hatching in the residual yolk.

The fact that maternal transfer involves specific antibody has been demonstrated for tetanus antitoxin, diphtheria antitoxin, neutralizing antibody to Newcastle disease virus, immunity to duck hepatitis, opsoniz-ing antibodies in the clearance of *Escherichia coli*, and many other anti-bodies to bacteria, protozoa and foreign proteins. Antiviral antibodies have been shown to be transferred in a variety of species including chickens, pigeons, sparrows, crows, swallows, herons and magpies. Immunity conferred upon the young by the mother often persists for about a month. It must be taken into account in programmes for immunizing poultry—just as for prophylactic immunization in mammals—since passively acquired antibody can interact with the antigen and thus inhibit stimulation of the infant's own immune system, e.g. passively transferred maternal antibody has been shown to interfere with immunization of chicks by live or formalin-inactivated Newcastle disease vaccines.

Onset of immunocompetence

The chick's own defence mechanisms are, of course, developing during embryonic life. In birds, as in poikilotherm larvae, macrophage function can be demonstrated very early in ontogeny. Uptake of particulate matter by the yolk sac occurs as early as the 3rd day of incubation, macrophages migrate into wound areas by day 7, and the embryonic liver is a phagocytic organ by day 10. Immunocompetence appears during the last week of incubation: transplantation immunity begins at about day 15, and is well developed by 2 days after hatching, while induction of humoral immune responses also starts at about the same time. Thus injection of goat erythrocytes on the 15th day of incubation leads to the production of opsonizing antibody which can be demonstrated one week later by its effect on immune clearance of the antigen. Some newly-hatched chicks and practically all week-old birds are capable of producing agglutinating antibody to foreign erythrocytes.

8.1.7. *Lymphoid tissues*

The primary lymphoid system of birds is unique in that the thymus-independent lineage of immune cells (the B-cells) differentiate in a special organ peculiar to birds, the bursa of Fabricius (often simply referred to as 'the bursa'). The thymus plays its usual role in the development of T-cells. Among the secondary lymphoid organs, the spleen is architecturally the most complex. The lymph nodes are relatively simple structures compared with those of mammals (see figure 8.5 and figure 9.2). Other lymphoid tissues include the oesophageal and pharyngeal tonsils, the caecal tonsils (which are a pair of diverticula from the ilio-colic region of the gut) and Harder's glands of the orbit (figure 8.2). In addition, there is much diffuse tissue in the form of infiltrating lymphocytes and solitary lymphoid nodules in a wide range of organs including the intestinal wall, the skin, the walls of lymphatic vessels, the periportal tissue of the liver, the gonads, pancreas and other internal organs. The bone marrow is haemopoietic and produces both granulocytes and lymphocytes.

The thymus

Ontogenetic development. In birds the thymus is an elongated lobulated gland, usually with seven lobes on each side, lying in the neck alongside the jugular veins. It arises from the 3rd and 4th pharyngeal pouches and,

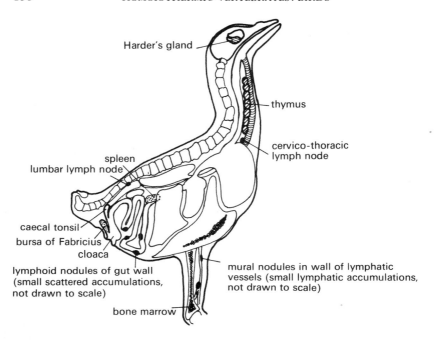

Figure 8.2.   Lymphoid organs of a bird
In addition to the major lymphoid organs shown, birds possess a
large amount of diffuse lymphoid tissue—in the gut wall, in the walls of
lymphatic vessels, in the skin, and in other organs. This is indicated
in the diagram in a few of its sites only, and it is drawn to an enlarged
scale. The lymph nodes figured in the diagram are not found in all
species of birds, e.g. they are absent in the chicken. Where avian
lymph nodes occur, there may be up to six pairs.

as in other vertebrates, ectoderm/endoderm interactions play an
important part in its induction. In the chick it is the ectoderm of the
dorsal part of the pouch region which differentiates to form the epithelial
thymic bud. The bud appears on the fifth day of incubation and has
separated from the pharyngeal epithelium by the 6th day. Between days
7 and 8 a new cell type appears which is probably the precursor of the
thymic lymphoid cells. Its origin has been a matter of much debate.
Several histological and *in vitro* studies (in mammals as well as in birds)
support the theory that lymphoid cells differentiate from the epithelial
elements of the thymic rudiment, but experiments in which the migrations

of labelled cells are followed suggest an extra-thymic origin. Such experiments have been done in the chicken by establishing yolk sac anastomoses at the 4th or 5th day of incubation. If one parabiont is a female, the other a male, their respective cells can be traced by the sex chromosome marker, the female having a large Z and a smaller W chromosome, while the male has a pair of the large ZZ form. When the parabiont embryos were sampled on the 14th to 16th day of incubation, up to half of the dividing cells in the thymus were found to be derived from the partner; i.e. there appeared to be an inflow of cells into the developing organ. Further experiments in which thymic rudiments were cultured *in vitro*, or grown as explants on the chorio-allantoic membrane, demonstrated the inability of the thymus of the 6-day-old chick to become a lymphoid organ if deprived of the normal ingress of precursor cells whereas, under similar circumstances, differentiation of lymphoid cells could occur in older thymic buds, which presumably had already acquired their immigrant precursor cells.

The early embryonic history of the stem cells which enter the thymus is unknown. It has been suggested that the yolk sac (which gives rise to multipotential haemopoietic cells *in situ*) is the immediate contributor, since this is the only major haemopoietic organ present in such young embryos. From this it seems that the processes which initially establish the thymus as a primary lymphoid organ (namely, entry of haemopoietic stem cells) are similar to those which maintain a working system in the adult mammal where influx of blood-borne stem cells into the thymus has been demonstrated using chromosome markers; in the adult mammal they come from the bone marrow. These experiments, in which labelled cells are externally applied, should be reconciled with findings in anurans where the label is within the thymic rudiment itself (see section 6.1.5), since vertebrates are unlikely to differ in anything as fundamental as the origin of their thymic lymphocytes. It is possible that immigrant cells interact with the epithelial cells, rather than give rise to lymphocytes themselves, but the answers may well lie in the different designs of the experiments which are looking at complex patterns of cell movements and differentiation processes at different points in the sequence.

Lymphoid stem cells proliferate rapidly within the thymus from about the 9th to 10th day of incubation, and a well-defined cortex and medulla is established by day 12. The thymus is a large organ in the young bird, but after about the second or third month it begins to shrink in size. However, unlike the irreversible process of age involution in a mammal, post-puberal regression of the thymus in birds shows seasonal recovery.

Thus the thymus in a number of avian species regains its enlarged size and juvenile histology for some weeks following at least the first sexual cycle. This is probably mediated through the endocrine system.

Role of the thymus. The role of the avian thymus in cell-mediated immunity is very similar to that in mammals, and many of the functions of mammalian T-cells are paralleled in birds. Migration of chicken thymic cells to secondary lymphoid organs, such as the spleen and caecal tonsils, has been demonstrated using radioactive markers; early thymectomy reduces the number of lymphocytes in these organs and in the peripheral blood. Thymectomy also diminishes the ability of the animal's lymphocytes to induce graft-versus-host reactions and to respond to stimulation by phytohaemagglutinin (PHA). The survival of skin allografts is prolonged in thymectomized birds, and delayed hypersensitivity responses are suppressed. The latter response is usually tested routinely by the wattle reaction (figure 8.3). In this test the bird is immunized, and at a later date challenged with the same antigen by intradermal injection into one wattle. A positive reaction (which is present in normal birds but absent after thymectomy) involves infiltration of the injection area with lymphocytes, macrophages and other cells, and causes obvious swelling.

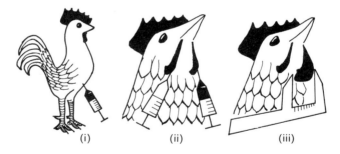

(i)   (ii)   (iii)

Figure 8.3.   Delayed hypersensitivity responses in the chicken
In birds the wattle is used as a site for delayed hypersensitivity reactions. The animal is immunized (i), and after a suitable period (e.g. about four weeks) injected again with the same antigen, this time by intradermal administration into one wattle (ii). The other wattle receives a control injection. After 24 hours, the thickness of both wattles is measured (iii). In a positive reaction the wattle on the antigen-stimulated side shows obvious swelling (e.g. to some three times the size of that receiving the control injection). Histologically there is infiltration with lymphocytes, macrophages and other cells. Similar tests for delayed hypersensitivity reactions can employ other sites, e.g. the foot pad of the rat.

Lymphokine factors have been investigated in birds, and the avian mitogenic factor has been found to be thymus-dependent. This is a soluble agent released by stimulated T-cells which acts in a non-specific way to stimulate proliferation of other lymphocytes. Thymectomy in birds, as in mammals, enhances both the growth of tumours and the number of "takes". Thymus-dependent surveillance has been demonstrated in the chicken in relation to diseases caused by oncogenic (tumour-inducing) viruses.

Attempts to demonstrate a role of the thymus in antibody production in chickens have been hampered by difficulties in obtaining good depletion of T-cells. Thus thymectomy is notoriously difficult in the bird because the lower thymic lobes are nearly always firmly attached to vital structures in the upper mediastinum. This led to equivocal results in some of the earlier experiments. Sometimes thymectomy is combined with irradiation in an attempt to deplete peripheral T-cells. Recently, however, antisera have been developed which react specifically against thymus cells in chickens and, if these are used in neonatally thymectomized birds, they help to knock out the T-cells more completely. In these experiments an adverse effect on antibody production to some antigens could be demonstrated (e.g. to foreign erythrocytes) while with other antigens, such as killed *Brucella abortus* organisms, antibody production was relatively unaffected. Thus in birds, as in other vertebrates, T-cells are necessary for full expression of the humoral immune response. They can be shown to act synergistically with B-cells in experiments in which the bird is rendered immunologically incompetent (by cyclophosphamide treatment plus irradiation) and then restored by injection of competent cells. If either thymus cells or bursa cells are given alone, neither will restore the immune response to foreign erythrocytes but, if T-cells are given together with B-cells, they act synergistically to produce positive antibody responses (as T-cell "helper" cells do in similarly designed experiments in mammals).

Surface immunoglobulins are readily demonstrated by immuno-fluorescence methods on avian B-cells, but not on thymus cells. In this respect birds resemble mammals, and differ from some of the poikilotherms. However, recent techniques of surface radio-iodination, followed by extraction and specific immunological precipitation, have identified IgM immunoglobulin on thymus cells from newly-hatched chickens at a time when the only serum immunoglobulin present was maternally derived IgG. It is therefore suggested that surface-borne immunoglobulins probably act as antigen receptors on thymic cells as well as on B-cells.

Later in life, the avian thymus, in addition to being a primary lymphoid organ, also becomes a tissue in which B-lymphocytes occur. Radio-labelled bursa-derived cells can be traced to the thymus, as well as to peripheral lymphoid organs; plasma cells and germinal centres are found in the medulla, and thymic plaque-forming cells (PFCs) can be demonstrated in immunized birds. The plasma cells begin to appear in the thymus at about one month after hatching, and their numbers increase following antigenic stimulation. The thymus therefore partially assumes the role of a secondary lymphoid organ.

The bursa of Fabricius

Ontogenetic development. The bursa of Fabricius arises as a sac-like evagination of the dorsal wall of the cloaca, in a region where the endoderm of the cloaca is in contact with the ectoderm, i.e. like the thymus, it forms at a site of ectodermal/endodermal interactions. In the chicken, the anlage appears at the 5th day of incubation. The bursal wall develops longitudinal folds, and by the 12th day these proliferate small epithelial buds (figure 8.4). The buds subsequently undergo lymphoid transformation, commencing on day 12–13. The origin of the lymphoid cells in the bursa of Fabricius is a matter of debate, but macrochromosomal studies on parabiosed male and female embryos similar to those described on p. 139 suggest that in the bursa, as in the thymus, the lymphoid cell precursors are derived from immigrant blood-borne stem cells. These are probably of yolk-sac origin. The yolk sac is the first haemopoietic organ to develop, and its cells are probably multipotential, as evidenced by their ability to repopulate both lymphoid and other blood-forming tissues of irradiated embryos.

It has been suggested that the primary lymphoid organs not only have an essential inductive influence on these stem cells, but also that their epithelium profoundly influences later functional development: if they lodge in the thymus they may differentiate along the T-cell lineage; if they lodge in the bursa they can become B-cells. From the 14–15th day onwards, the stem cells give rise to lymphocytes. Each follicle within the bursa develops a richly lymphocytic mantle which resembles the cortex of the thymus; it is usually outermost, although in the ostrich, the rhea and various birds of prey the 'cortex' may be centrally located. The bursa is a lymphocytic organ by the time of hatching, the bursa and the thymus being the only fully differentiated lymphoid organs at this time. The bursa reaches its maximum size in about the 2nd to 3rd month but, at the onset of sexual maturity, it regresses and in older birds disappears completely—unlike the thymus which persists as a small atrophic organ. Thus the bursa shows the characteristics of a primary lymphoid organ in (*a*) its early differentiation, (*b*) the intimate association between lymphocytes and epithelial cells, (*c*) its high level of proliferative activity which seems to be independent of antigenic stimulation, and (*d*) its susceptibility to age involution. Also, like the thymus, the bursa shows hormonally mediated involution during stress.

Role of the bursa. The discovery that the bursa is a primary lymphoid organ concerned with the differentiation of antibody-forming cell precursors (B-cells) dates from the mid-1950s, when it was found that surgical removal of the bursa from hatchlings (but not from older birds) suppressed the ability of the animal to make specific antibodies when immunized with *Salmonella typhimurium O* antigen. These initial experi-

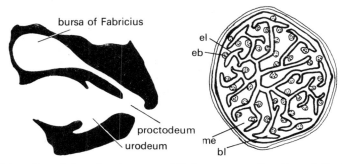

(*a*) sagittal section of cloacal region   (*b*) transverse section through the bursa
                                                         at 14 days of incubation

Figure 8.4. Development of the bursa of Fabricius of the chicken
(*a*) Development of the bursa as a dorsal diverticulum from the posterior cloacal wall.
(*b*) Transverse section through the embryonic bursa at the 14th day of incubation. Nodular thickenings (epithelial buds (eb)) appear in the epithelium (el) which lines the bursa lumen (bl). These buds sink into the surrounding connective tissue, but still retain contact with the bursal epithelium, which itself is continuous with the bursal duct and cloaca. The epithelial bud later fills with proliferating lymphocytes. Lymphoid cells also appear in the surrounding mesenchymatous tissue (me).
From Jolly, J. (1915), "La bourse de Fabricius et les organes lympho-épithéliaux", *Archives d'anatomie microscopique*, **16**, 363–547 (with modifications).

ments were followed by extensive studies on bursectomized birds in a number of laboratories. The bursa is usually removed at as early an age as possible, and in some experiments surgical bursectomy is combined with irradiation. It was also found that testosterone treatment during embryogenesis, either by dipping the egg at day 3 or injecting the embryo during the early stages of bursal development, suppresses bursal function; this can be made more effective by treating the bird with cyclophosphamide after hatching to further inhibit any B-cell precursors.

Both chemical bursectomy of this kind and early surgical bursectomy will render a proportion of the treated birds completely agammaglobulinaemic, i.e. they produce neither specific antibody nor serum immunoglobulins, both IgM and IgG being suppressed. Their lymphoid organs lack germinal centres and plasma cells, and they fail to produce plaque-forming cells (PFCs) after immunization. On the other hand, the T-cell system remains intact, and the bursectomized bird responds normally to allografts and in delayed hypersensitivity reactions. The circulating small lymphocytes are present in normal numbers; they show mitogenic responses to phytohaemagglutinin (PHA) and they are effective in graft-versus-host reactions.

In the chick, the proportion of bursal cells which bear immunoglobulin on their surface is high (higher than in any mammalian organs). The bursal cells can synthesize immunoglobulin from a very early stage of development. This has been shown by sensitive *in vitro* culture tests and by immunofluorescent staining. Indeed the latter technique, using goat antibodies to chicken immunoglobulin μ-chains, γ-chains and light chains, has detected IgM synthesis by bursal cells as soon as recognizable lymphocytes appear in the bursa, i.e. at about the 14th day of incubation. IgG-producing cells are found later, at around the time of hatching. IgM is the first class of immunoglobulin which can be detected in ontogeny, and it has been suggested that even cells which will eventually produce IgG or IgA, initially express IgM on their surface. The fact that "partial", or relatively late, bursectomy can suppress IgG production without affecting IgM synthesis has been explained by suggesting that some cells synthesizing IgM were already in the peripheral tissues before the bursa was destroyed, but were unable to switch to IgG production in the absence of the bursa. Thus the bursa is seen as a site of maturation of stem cells to B-lymphocytes which possess surface immunoglobulin "receptors" and which are committed both to the class and specificity of their immunoglobulin product.

Entry of radio-labelled bursal cells into the secondary lymphoid organs has been demonstrated in a number of experiments, and it is thought that most antigenic stimulation takes place in these peripheral tissues. Thus, although plasma cells can be found within the bursa, they are mainly under the epithelium rather than in the bursal follicles, and injection of antigen by most routes fails to elicit antibody production in the bursa itself. An exception occurs if antigen is administered from the cloaca via the bursal duct. In this case antibody production by bursal cells could be demonstrated to an enteric form of *Escherichia coli*, suggesting that the bursa may perhaps play a direct role in immunity to local infections.

Under normal circumstances the bursa is probably the sole source of immunocompetent B-cells. A few experiments suggest the possibility of alternative pathways however. Thus birds in which the tail area, with the presumptive bursal region, was amputated in the 70-hour-old embryo, still produced a little immunoglobulin; also chemical bursectomy by testosterone treatment during early embryogenesis has little effect on IgM synthesis. Furthermore, in chemically bursectomized birds in a batch where antibody production was suppressed in some of the birds but not in others, no trace of a bursa could be found even in the responsive birds. Surface immunoglobulins have been detected on yolk-sac cells in the 12-day-old embryo; it is possible that in the absence of the bursa some of these cells may still be capable of a limited amount of B-cell line differentiation elsewhere in the body.

It is interesting that in bursectomized irradiated chickens which are completely agammaglobulinaemic (possessing neither IgM nor IgG), a protein has been described in the serum which is apparently made up of only heavy (μ) chains of IgM. This is very similar to the "heavy chain only" immunoglobulin of the lamprey. This immunoglobulin-like protein may be a primordial form synthesized either independently of the bursa, or as an early product before immunocompetent cells are sufficiently differentiated to produce IgM.

The spleen

In the chick embryo the splenic anlage appears on the 8th day of incubation as a mesenchymal condensation interspersed with vascular spaces. By the end of the incubation period, the future white pulp can be distinguished from the red pulp, and it becomes increasingly lymphocytic during the first week post-hatching. The splenic lymphoid cells accumulate in special locations in relation to the vasculature to form (a) lymphocytic cuffs surrounding the central arterioles—these are depleted of lymphocytes in thymectomized animals and are generally regarded as a thymus-dependent component; (b) lymphoid cells surrounding the Schweigger-Seidel sheaths (i.e. the tissue which sheaths arterioles before they terminate in the red pulp)— these lymphoid cells are slightly pyroninophilic, they resemble cells of the mammalian marginal zone (figure 1.13) and are part of the bursa-dependent system; (c) the germinal centres.

As in the mammal, the germinal centres are functionally concerned with expansion of the B-cell population involved in immunoglobulin synthesis, but they differ structurally from mammalian germinal centres in that in the bird the germinal centre lacks a lymphocytic corona and is more definitely delineated by encircling connective tissue. Germinal centre formation in the avian spleen is related to antigen-trapping. Radio-labelled soluble protein antigen (^{125}I-human serum albumin) has been shown to enter the spleen at the periphery of the Schweigger-Seidel sheaths, probably in the form of antigen/antibody complexes, thence to be transported by dendritic cells through the white pulp, following alongside the penicillary (sheathed) arterioles to their point of origin from the central arteriole. During this migration the antigen-bearing dendritic cells appear to capture and accumulate lymphocytes, presumably those which have receptors corresponding to the antigen; subsequent pyroninophilic transformation and mitoses of these lymphocytes produce a recognizable germinal centre in which trapped antigen can be demonstrated on the dendritic processes of the antigen-bearing cells.

The presence of the bursa in the early post-hatching period is essential for germinal centre development. Radio-labelled bursal cells can be traced to the germinal centres, and cells from the bursa are capable of restoring germinal centre formation in animals depleted by cyclophosphamide treatment or by bursectomy. In older chickens, cells from the secondary lymphoid organs also become capable of effecting reconstitution; cells from the spleen are able to do so by week 3, those from the bone marrow by week 6. Furthermore in the 20-month-old bird where the bursa has involuted, germinal centres are still formed in response to antigenic stimulation, in the spleen and in other secondary lymphoid organs, albeit more slowly and to a lesser extent than in younger animals. Cells involved in germinal centre formation in the chicken are therefore not necessarily derived by direct migration from the bursa to the spleen; after the early developmental period they may be housed elsewhere. The spleen gains in relative importance for antibody production as the animal gets older, and splenectomy has more effect on the antibody response to BSA (bovine serum albumin) in 4-month-old chickens than in younger birds.

Other lymphoid organs

In recent years it has become possible to analyse the components of the secondary lymphoid organs of the chicken in terms of their T-cell and B-cell populations, using antiserum specifically directed against thymus cells or against bursal cells. These antisera are raised in another species (e.g. rabbit or turkey), cross-absorbed to get rid of unwanted activities, and either tagged for use in immunofluorescence studies, or used with complement in cytotoxicity tests. These studies confirm the presence of a small percentage of B-cells in the thymus. They also indicate that in the bone marrow about a quarter of the white-cell population of one-day-old chickens bears the B-cell-marker, although only a few of these cells have demonstrable surface-associated immunoglobulin.

The lymph nodes of birds arise from proliferations in the wall of lymphatic vessels. During development, small buds of mesenchymatous tissue project into the lumen, and these fuse together to enclose lymphatic sinusoids, while the main lumen of the lymph vessel remains as the central sinus (figure 8.5). Germinal centres develop in the lymphoid tissue next to the central sinus, while the "medulla" is peripheral. The avian lymph node has no external capsule, and blood vessels penetrate the cords of lymphoid tissue at several points, rather than through a single hilus. This is a different arrangement from that of the mammalian lymph node (figure 9.2) with its outer sinus and peripheral cortex, and the avian lymph node is considerably less complex architecturally. Where lymph nodes occur in birds,

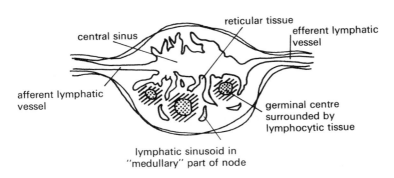

Figure 8.5. Lymph node of a bird
The avian lymph node has a central sinus which represents the main lumen of a lymphatic vessel. Germinal centres develop in the lymphoid tissue around this central sinus. Most of the "medullary" tissue lies towards the periphery of the node.

it is usual to find a pair of lumbar nodes, and a pair of nodes in the cervico-thoracic region, although others may also be present. The chicken lacks these structures, but lymphatic nodules occur in the walls of its lymphatic vessels (mural nodules). These are found regularly in the vessels of the neck, wing and hindlimb, and they frequently show germinal centres.

Harder's gland of the orbit is a lymphoid organ in birds. Cells with demonstrable surface immunoglobulin can be demonstrated within it in the 3-week-old chick. Their numbers rise rapidly and plasma cells are plentiful. The secretion from this gland (which washes the nictitating membrane) discharges from the orbit via the lachrymal ducts and eventually may be swallowed from the mouth. The lachrymal ducts also show scattered lymphoid nodules.

Extensive lymphoid areas occur in the caecal tonsils, and plasma cells may be found in large numbers in these organs. The caecal tonsils are well developed in the two-month-old chicken, and by 4 months of age they are populated with many cells which bear surface immunoglobulin. Diffuse lymphoid accumulations occur in the skin; their cells have been shown to be immunocompetent by their ability to elicit graft-versus-host reactions. Small lymphoid nodules are also found scattered in the intestinal tract. In germ-free chickens, this type of lymphoid tissue which is in contact with the bacterial flora contains considerably fewer lymphocytes than in conventionally reared animals. It is suggested that the presence of micro-organisms in the gut lumen may be a major stimulus to the development of the germinal centres and plasma cells in the lymphoid tissues of the gut wall.

8.2. Conclusions

The birds are an advanced group with an active way of life and a high body temperature. In such animals we might expect to find an efficient and specialized immune system. Comparison with the other class of homoiothermic animals (the mammals) should reveal both homologies and convergent evolution, as well as special adaptations, for it is some 300 million years since the reptilian ancestors of the birds separated from those of mammalian stock. It seems that in the immune system of birds and mammals much is homologous at the cellular level; at the tissue level there is some divergence, while other aspects, such as the status of the avian major histocompatibility system and the origins of the secretory antibody of birds, require further investigation.

A unique avian specialization is the bursa of Fabricius. Functional delineation of the B-cell and T-cell lines, and special microenvironments for their differentiation, occur in other vertebrate groups, but it is only in birds that the site of primary differentiation of B-lineage cells becomes isolated into an anatomically distinct organ. This may well be a recent adaptation, albeit one which possibly emphasizes pre-existing potentialities of the gut epithelium. There may be a special need in birds to hasten and amplify B-cell differentiation in order to defend the warm-blooded but relatively unprotected (i.e. non-suckled) chick; thus the baby bird may need to bring its defences into play very rapidly after hatching, particularly in relation to its intake via the gastro-intestinal tract. Whatever the reasons for this new development, and whatever the relationships to the so-called "bursa-equivalents" elsewhere, in practical terms the separation of B-cell and T-cell lineages in the bird provides an extremely important model. Only in the bursectomized bird can we readily obtain a "T-cell animal", i.e. one in which the B-cell population is convincingly depleted while the T-cell system remains intact.

CHAPTER NINE

HOMOIOTHERMIC VERTEBRATES: MAMMALS

9.1. Mammalia

Mammals have provided the yardstick for our comparative studies throughout the book and their immune system forms the basis of much of Chapter 1. In the present chapter therefore we make no attempt to review the entire field of mammalian immunology; we simply concentrate on some of the more interesting evolutionary aspects within the class.

Mammals first appear in the Triassic. They are descendants of the synapsid reptiles, a group whose divergence from other reptilian stocks occurred far back in the Carboniferous period. The monotremes (Prototheria) technically qualify for classification as mammals but also retain a number of reptilian features including the habit of egg-laying. They are represented only by the platypus and the echidnas and their evolutionary history is unknown. The marsupials (Metatheria) and the placental mammals (Eutheria) are obviously more advanced. Both are viviparous; the extra-embryonic membranes which first arose in the amniote egg acquire a new relationship with the maternal tissues in marsupial and eutherian mammals, a relationship which has significant immunological implications.

Marsupials and eutherians separated in the Cretaceous period, some 100 million years ago, having arisen from a group of Mesozoic mammals known as the Pantotheria (figure 7.1). In marsupials gestation is short and the young are born at a very immature stage of development. They are then carried by the mother for a further period, usually in a special pouch. The marsupial "pouch young" are useful models for studies on the early exposure to various forms of antigenic stimulation and on the effects of "foetal" thymectomy since they are readily accessible in the pouch at a stage when the eutherian foetus is still in the uterus. The North American opossum *Didelphis virginiana* is a primitive marsupial which shows little change from its Cretaceous ancestor and is an interesting representative of the early mammalian condition. Adaptive radiation from this early marsupial stock, occurring mainly in geographical isolation, has led to many examples of convergent evolution between the marsupials and the eutherians. The latter are the dominant group of present-day mammals; they are highly advanced vertebrates displaying varied specializations in the different eutherian orders.

9.1.1. *Transplantation reactions*

Alloimmune reactivity

The transplantation antigens of mammals present examples of genetic polymorphism of bewildering complexity. Alloantigen systems are well documented for mice, rats and man, and there are also studies on rabbits, dogs and a number of other domestic animals. The ready availability of inbred lines of mice has been of particular importance in helping to unravel the genetics in terms of both blood group and histocompatibility systems. As we have already discussed for chickens (section 8.1.1), one major histocompatibility locus predominates in terms of the sensitizing potency of its products. In the mouse this is the H-2 locus. Following the discovery of the H-2, a number of additional loci controlling the production of a variety of blood group and tissue antigens has been described in mice. The major H-2 locus is extremely polymorphic; the 20 or so H-2 alleles identified in laboratory colonies inadequately reflect the large number of different H-2 alleles occurring in mice captured from the wild. A highly polymorphic genetic system also occurs in man and probably typifies transplantation systems in general. Selective pressure in favour of heterozygotes would help to maintain this allogeneic polymorphism. A survival advantage which occurs in foetuses possessing histocompatibility antigens absent from the mother may be an important factor here; this is discussed in the following section on maternal-foetal relationships.

Transplantation reactions have not been studied in monotremes. In other mammals grafts are rejected in an acute fashion and there is clear second-set memory. The median rejection time (MST) of first-set grafts exchanged across the major H-2 barrier of the mouse is about 10 days. In outbred adult opossums *Didelphis virginiana*, rejection takes 7–22 days while in the quokka *Setonix brachyurus* (a more advanced diprotodont marsupial) grafts are rejected within a fortnight (8–14 days). The process of graft rejection in the quokka is similar to that in the mouse; it involves cellular infiltration and later scab formation.

Frequently, although not always, the eutherian foetus or neonate once it is capable of rejecting a graft can do so with adult levels of reactivity. This is true for foetal sheep which start to display efficient alloimmune responses at 70 days before birth (the gestation period is 147 days). In marsupials cell-mediated immune responses develop more gradually. Thus in the opossum *Didelphis virginiana*, juveniles aged three months or more show acute rejection of maternal skin but if similar grafts are placed on 17-day-old pouch young their subsequent rejection is a chronic process which takes some 13 weeks for completion.

Foetal-maternal interactions

Viviparity is a method of reproduction which has evolved many times in vertebrates. It occurs in several families of chondrichthian fish (e.g. a number of sharks and rays), a few teleosts, some amphibians (e.g. viviparous salamanders) and several reptiles (various lizards and snakes). In none of these groups does the relationship between mother and foetus become as intimate as in the mammals, but all share the problem inherent in the relationship, namely that the young bear the status of an allograft in relation to the mother by virtue of the genetic moiety inherited from the father (see section 4.2.1).

The immunological implications of pregnancy have been extensively investigated in mammals but many questions remain unanswered. As an allograft the foetus would seem liable to rejection. It is known to be capable of expressing transplantation antigens and the mother of responding to them. It has even been suggested that immunological reactions assist implantation and may be essential for securement of the blastocyst through a local inflammatory reaction. The fact that implantation can occur successfully in highly inbred strains argues against this theory, although tissue-specific antigens or residual heterozygosity could still be involved.

In many mammalian species, including laboratory rodents and man, the wall of the blastocyst proliferates immediately after implantation, and the resulting trophoblast invades the uterine mucosa. At this stage and in the established placenta there is intimate contact of histoincompatible elements, namely the trophoblast of the foetus and the uterine tissues of the mother. It has been suggested that the trophoblast cells are protected by a lining of fibrinoid-like material which places a physical barrier between the mother and foetus. However it is known that cells can cross the placenta. Entry of foetal cells into the maternal circulation may perhaps elicit the production of enhancing antibodies and favour specific maternal non-reactivity. Entry in the other direction of maternal lymphocytes into the foetus has also been demonstrated. Their potentially injurious effects are probably counteracted by the immune competence of the foetus itself; indeed, these may be the first pathogens which it encounters.

Despite these considerations, antigenic differences are certainly not without effect; the adverse consequences of rhesus blood group incompatibility in man, for example, are well known. A more favourable outcome of antigenic disparity has recently been suggested whereby immune interaction between maternal cells and an antigenically incompatible foetus may actually increase the survival chances of such offspring. This follows from the observation in rats and mice that if one inbred strain is mated with another inbred strain, the resulting hybrid foetus is larger than a pure-bred foetus from either parental line and is supported by a heavier placenta. It is suggested that the immune response of the maternal cells to paternally derived histocompatibility antigens of the hybrid foetus may result in this more vascular placenta which is larger by up to 20%. Involvement of the immune system in the reaction is substantiated by its increase when the mother is made immune to paternal tissues and its reduction when she is made tolerant to them. The selective advantage to foetuses which are unlike the mother could be a factor which helps to maintain balanced polymorphism at the major histocompatibility loci.

9.1.2. Humoral immunity in mammals

Antibody production

Antibody production has been studied in the echidna *Tachyglossus aculeatus*. These monotremes synthesize both IgM and IgG antibody. The primary response to immunization with *Salmonella adelaide* flagella is similar to that in eutherian mammals both in its kinetics and in the total amount of antibody produced, although IgG does not completely replace the IgM in all animals. Echidnas show immunological memory in antibody production but their secondary responses to *Salmonella adelaide* flagellae are considerably weaker than those of eutherian mammals.

In marsupials good secondary responses can be demonstrated. The secondary antibody levels are well in excess of the primary titres and they yield predominantly IgG. Nevertheless certain features of the marsupial humoral response remain intermediate between the condition in eutherian mammals and that in poikilothermic vertebrates. These include the persistence of IgM and the slow conversion of IgM to IgG in the primary responses of both quokkas and opossums. Thus a common pattern in eutherian mammals is for IgM to appear after a relatively short latent period, to peak in the second week and then decline giving way to IgG, whereas in opossums the reaction proceeds more slowly and it takes some 3 to 4 weeks before both IgM and IgG are found in the serum. This time course is more like that of a poikilothermic vertebrate, although in hyperimmunized opossums the conversion from IgM to IgG may be quicker and more complete.

Another similarity to many poikilotherms is the relatively poor reaction of the opossum to soluble antigens such as bovine serum albumin (BSA) as compared with good responses to particulate antigens, for example those of bacteria and viruses. Titres in the opossum remain somewhat lower than those of eutherian mammals but in the advanced diprotodont marsupials responses to particulate antigens are quite strong with respectable levels of antibody production. This has been shown for the quokka *Setonix brachyurus*, the tammar *Macropus eugenii* and the Australian (diprotodont) opossum *Trichosurus vulpecula*. In these marsupials part of the low-molecular-weight antibody was found to be 2-mercaptoethanol-sensitive; this is not peculiar to marsupials however (see section 1.4.2).

The primitive North American opossum *Didelphis virginiana* appears to be somewhat deficient in its delayed hypersensitivity reactions as well as in its humoral antibody responses; for example it shows only minimal cutaneous reactions to tuberculin. It is therefore of interest to know the immune capabilities of the more primitive orders of the other major branch—the eutherian mammals.

Primitive eutherians include the Order Insectivora whose members (hedgehogs, shrews, etc.) remain close to the ancestral condition; also the bats (order Chiroptera) which are probably related to insectivore stock. Information on these animals stems mainly from epidemiological surveys of diseases in which they are potential carriers of organisms pathogenic to man or his domestic animals. This applies particularly to bats as a possible reservoir of viral infections. Experimental immunization in bats shows their reactions to be relatively inefficient. For example, the response of the big brown bat *Eptesicus fuscus* to viral antigens (bacteriophage) is initially quite rapid, but the magnitude and duration of antibody production is less than in common laboratory mammals, and more of the antibody remains in the 2-mercaptoethanol-sensitive fraction.

Effect of temperature

Mammals are homoiotherms and any influence of environmental temperature on immune responses is more likely to occur via hormonally-mediated stress reactions than in a direct way. However, some mammals hibernate and here temperature may have a more direct effect. In the big brown bat *Eptesicus fuscus* it has been shown that ambient temperature affects both body temperature and metabolic rate. These creatures form neutralizing antibody to Japanese B encephalitis virus more readily at ambient temperatures of 37 °C than at 24 °C, and no antibody production occurs in infected animals maintained for prolonged periods at 8 °C. At 8 °C active virus persists in the tissues of the dormant animal, a finding which is relevant to the potential harbouring of viral pathogens by infected bats during the winter season.

The effect of temperature on humoral immunity in hibernating mammals is in some ways similar to that in poikilotherms, since early events in the immunization process can occur at low temperature. Thus hibernating ground squirrels *Citellus tridecemlineatus* immunized in the cold produce circulating antibody to sheep erythrocytes within a few days of arousal from hibernation, in contrast to the usual latent period of over a week for a primary immune response. When animals which had already given a primary response before hibernating are reinjected shortly after arousal, antibody appears after a short latent period typical of the secondary reaction but it fails to reach high titres; i.e. processes leading to the production of secondary levels of circulating antibody are inhibited during hibernation. It is also of interest that ground squirrels maintained at 22–24 °C still show seasonal variation in their immune responses.

Immunoglobulin classes

In addition to the IgM and IgG immunoglobulins, man and perhaps most eutherians, can synthesize IgA, IgD and IgE. It now seems that IgA and IgE at least are also present in marsupials, together with the IgM and IgG classes. In monotremes only IgM and IgG have been detected. Analyses of echidna IgG reveal a striking resemblance to the IgG of man. The heavy chains (γ-chains) show close similarities in their electrophoretic mobilities and other properties and there is a degree of immunological cross-reactivity between echidna IgG and human IgG. Thus monotremes appear to be the first group to express a γ-chain gene directly homo-logous to the γ-chain gene of man, since there is reason to believe that the γ-chain of non-mammalian vertebrates is not strictly homologous to that of human IgG (see section 6.1.4).

IgG is the dominant immunoglobulin class in mammals. Subclasses occur within this class in both eutherians and marsupials. Eutherians, in particular, show a considerable complexity of immunoglobulins including subclasses of IgM and IgA as well as of IgG. In diprotodont marsupials (quokkas, tammars and Australian opossums) a low-molecular-weight class has been identified which is synthesized separately from IgM and IgG. This is tentatively placed in the heterogeneous group of IgN-like low-molecular-weight immunoglobulins along with those of lungfish, turtles, ducks, rabbits and other species.

IgA has been identified in at least 6 orders of eutherian mammals where it plays a special protective role at mucosal surfaces and in external secretions in a number of species including man, rabbits, rodents, sheep, sea-lions, dogs and dolphins—a sufficiently wide range to suggest that it is universal in the eutherian line. Immunoglobulin molecules resembling IgA have also been identified in the diprotodont marsupial *Setonix brachyurus* (the quokka). They are antigenically distinct from the other immuno-globulin classes of the quokka (IgG_1, IgG_2 and IgM). Quokka IgA is present in low concentration in the serum and it is the major immuno-globulin in secretions such as tears, milk, urine and gut contents. More-over local antigenic stimulation of the mammary gland in lactating quokkas induces an antibody secretion into the milk which is restricted to the IgA class. Further structural information is required to ascertain whether quokka IgA is homologous to the IgA of eutherian mammals; no secretory piece has yet been found in marsupials.

Antibodies apparently homologous to the IgE of man occur in monkeys, rats, dogs and rabbits, while IgE-like activity in immediate hypersensitivity reactions has also been reported in mice, cows, sheep, pigs and quokkas. This suggests a widespread occurrence of the IgE-like class within the Mammalia.

Immediate hypersensitivity reactions

In some mammals immediate hypersensitivities are mediated by a subclass of IgG, such as the IgG_1 of guinea pigs. If these antibodies are passively transferred they remain fixed to the recipient's skin for a few days only. If the recipient is challenged with specific antigen, the hypersensitivity reaction involving mast-cell degranulation (passive cutaneous anaphylaxis) is of greatest magnitude if the antigen is injected within 2–6 hours (i.e.

both the persistence and the latent period of the reaction are short). This type of response can also occur in vertebrates other than mammals (e.g. in birds, see section 8.1.5).

Reaginic (IgE-mediated) immediate hypersensitivities, on the other hand, have so far been reported only in mammals. In these reactions the IgE may remain fixed to tissue receptors, probably on mast cells, for up to 6 weeks and the latent period for passive cutaneous anaphylaxis is more than 24 hours. It is interesting that in quokkas immediate hypersensitivities involve antibody which persists at skin sites for more than 10 days and for which the latent period in passive cutaneous anaphylaxis is 48–72 hours. Also, like IgE, the quokka antibody is inactivated by heating at 56 °C and by 2-mercaptoethanol treatment. Thus IgE-like antibodies may well date back to the pantothere ancestors of the marsupial and eutherian mammals. It has been suggested that IgE aids in the expulsion of metazoan parasites (and possibly of tumours). Various antibodies have been implicated in such mechanisms in lower vertebrates, even the IgM of urodeles (see section 5.1.1). Possibly IgE is a more sophisticated mammalian specialization, perhaps more intimately linked to mast cell functions.

9.1.3. Ontogeny of immunity

Transfer of maternal antibodies

The close relationship between mother and young in mammals provides plentiful opportunities for the transfer of maternal antibody to the young during pregnancy and lactation; in fact, however, this transfer usually takes place over a relatively restricted period. In man, monkeys, guinea pigs and rabbits all the antibody which appears in the serum of the young is transmitted before birth; in man and monkeys this occurs by way of the placenta, in guinea pigs and rabbits by passage across the yolk sac. In contrast, in artiodactyls (cattle, sheep, goats and pigs), in horses and in the diprotodont marsupials (quokkas), there is no transmission during the prenatal period; transfer of maternal antibody takes place instead by way of the secretions of the mammary glands. Rats, mice, hedgehogs, cats and dogs show an intermediate condition with transmission both before and after birth, maternal antibody being acquired by the foetus via the foetal membranes (placenta in dogs, yolk sac in rats and mice), also post-natally by the suckling animal.

Since mammary glands occur only in mammals (they are the diagnostic feature which gives the class its name) the passage of antibody to the suckling young is an evolutionary innovation. The first mammary gland secretion which the new-born animal receives (colostrum) plays an important role in the passive transfer of immunity. In artiodactyls (cattle, goats, sheep and pigs) the antibody titre of the colostrum of immunized mothers is equal to, or exceeds, that of the serum. This antibody is rapidly transferred to the suckling young whose own serum levels may soon come to equal those of the mammary gland secretion. In these animals the passage of immunoglobulin from the colostrum to the serum only takes place during a short period after birth; the capacity of the gut to absorb antibodies is soon lost and after 48 hours these immune proteins are digested and not transmitted. The protective value of antibody transferred in the mammary gland secretions is demonstrated by the high incidence of "scours" due to *Escherichia coli* which occurs when new-born calves are deprived of colostrum.

In contrast to the ungulates (artiodactyls and horses), passage of antibodies from the milk to the serum continues for some 16–20 days in suckling rats and mice and for up to 40 days in the hedgehog. In marsupials it is an even more extended process, possibly owing to the very immature state of development of the young marsupial at the time of birth. In quokkas, for example, antibody is passed via the milk to the serum of the pouch young for up to 6 months, i.e. until the young joey begins to leave the pouch and fend for itself. The quokka starts to take solid food before the absorption of antibody from the milk has ceased. In hedgehogs and opossums also, absorption continues after weaning has commenced. In the quokka, it is possible that milk by-passes the rumen but the mechanism whereby immunoglobulins escape digestion in the opossum and hedgehog is not fully understood.

The role of passively transferred maternal antibody is to provide immediate protection against ingress of micro-organisms during the initial period when the newborn enters an environment which is more highly pathogenic than that of the uterus. The maternal antibody in the serum of the young probably has its main function as an opsonizing antibody in helping to clear pathogenic micro-organisms in the initial infective phase; however, its presence can, under some circumstances, interfere with prophylactic immunization (see section 8.1.6). In most species the antibody concerned is predominantly IgG. Thus IgG is the only antibody which crosses the placental barrier to the foetus (e.g. in man). In rats, mice and quokkas, the intestinal wall can absorb IgG transferred in the milk but it excludes immunoglobulins of other classes. However in artiodactyls the intestinal wall is less selective and will transport IgM and IgA as well as IgG; so also will the yolk sac of the rabbit (Table 9.1).

Table 9.1. Passive transfer of maternal antibody to the offspring in vertebrates

Animal	Route of transfer	Class of immunoglobulin	
		IgG	IgM
man	placenta	+	−
rabbit	yolk sac	+	+
rat	yolk sac + colostrum	+	−
cattle	colostrum	+	+
quokka	colostrum	+	−
chick	yolk sac	+	−
			(+ via albumin)
amphibians and fish	(no definite evidence for transfer via yolk)		

The IgA which is present in mammary-gland secretions passes to the circulation of the young only in some species (e.g. artiodactyls); in others (e.g. man, rat) it is not transported across the intestinal wall. Maternal IgA may function mainly in the lumen of the alimentary tract. It appears to be more resistant than other immunoglobulins to digestion by proteolytic enzymes, perhaps by virtue of its secretory piece. It probably plays a protective role in helping to restrain ingress of pathogenic micro-organisms through the gut wall until such time as the cells of the lamina propria of the young animal are sufficiently antigenically stimulated to produce their own IgA antibody.

Onset of humoral immunocompetence

The placental barrier is remarkably specific in preventing micro-organisms from reaching the mammalian foetus; only a limited number of pathogens pass the barrier. However, the foetuses of mammals, especially those of large animals with long gestation periods, are frequently well able to respond immunologically in a positive way following antigenic stimulation, even though they may not normally be called upon to do so very often. On the other hand, large doses of antigen, particularly of experimentally administered allogeneic cells, may be tolerogenic in the immature mammal as in other vertebrates (see section 1.6.1).

From the experimental viewpoint, species which display transfer of immunity *in utero* are difficult subjects in which to investigate the immune capabilities of the young, because immunization can be complicated by the presence of maternal antibody. Better models are provided where there is no such transfer. For this reason the foetal sheep has been well investigated. In these animals production of antibody to bacteriophage can be demonstrated as early in gestation as is technically feasible to immunize and bleed the foetus (about 40 days), antibody to ferritin is elicited by 80 days, whereas humoral responses to ovalbumin do not occur until 120 days, and to heat-killed *Salmonella typhosa* not until after birth. Thus the maturation of immunocompetence appears to be antigen-dependent; perhaps this is due to step-wise differentiation of the effector cells, but it may depend upon other factors which affect antigenicity, or on the maturation of cells which co-operate in the response. Sheep at less than 80 days of gestation produce only IgM antibody, after this age IgG may also be synthesized. It seems that lack of maturity of the lymphoid tissues does not preclude the possibility of an immune response; in fact, some forms of antigenic stimulation can hasten histogenesis and differentiation to a level not normally seen in the lymphoid organs until after birth.

In marsupials immune capabilities develop more gradually. Marsupials are of interest because of their very immature condition at birth. The North American opossum when born after 12–13 days gestation is very small (only 0·01% of its adult weight) and it remains poikilothermic for the first two months of life. The marsupial-pouch young are, of course, well protected by the mother, and the maternal pouch secretions contain immunoglobulins which help to provide a defence against pathogens in the immediate environment of the young. In the opossum, antibody production to viral antigens can be elicited from as early as day 5 of pouch life, i.e. shortly after lymphocytes begin to appear in the thymus and lymph nodes (the thymus becomes lymphocytic at day 2 and the lymph nodes at day 3–6). Positive humoral responses to *Salmonella typhosa* flagellae first appear at day 8 and to the hapten determinant DNP (dinitrophenol) at day 15. IgM is most prominent in the response but IgG can also be detected. In marsupials, as in sheep, the competence to produce humoral antibody develops earlier than the ability to reject skin grafts. However, antibody titres in the immature period are considerably lower than those of older pouch young.

9.1.4. *Lymphoid tissues*

The monotremes (echidna) have a well-developed lymphoid system with thymus, spleen, chains of simple lymph nodes especially prominent in the cervical, axillary and pelvic regions, small mesenteric nodes, tonsils, appendix, Peyer's patches and bone marrow; germinal centres and plasma cells are well developed. These organs presumably date back to an early common ancestor in the synapsid reptiles, since they are possessed by mammals of all orders (see figure 9.1.).

The thymus

Anatomy and development. In the majority of mammals the entire thymus lies in the upper part of the thorax as it does in man. This is somewhat removed from the original vertebrate location. It reflects changes which

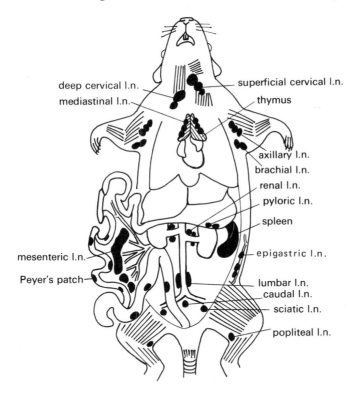

Figure 9.1.   Lymphoid organs of a mammal
Rat dissected to show the thymus, spleen, Peyer's patches, and the system of regional lymph nodes. Naming of the lymph nodes mainly follows that of Dunn, T. B. (1954), "Normal and Pathologic Anatomy of the Recticular Tissue in Laboratory Mice, with a Classification and Discussion of Neoplasms", *Journal of the National Cancer Institute*, **14**, 1281–1434.

occur during the formation of a distinct neck in land-living vertebrates, caudal migration of the thymus being more extensive in mammals than in other vertebrate classes. In some species, however, part or all of the thymus remains in the cervical region, and in this respect there are interesting parallels between marsupial and eutherian mammals. The thymus is cervical in position in the marsupial koalas and wombats and in eutherian guinea-pigs.

In the majority of diprotodont marsupials (e.g. quokkas) and in the eutherian degu *Octodon degu*, and in bats there is both a cervical and a thoracic organ, while the more primitive (polyprotodont) marsupials and most eutherian mammals have a thymus which lies wholly in the thoracic region. This scattered distribution may reflect the ancestral origin of the thymus from a position at the ectodermal/endodermal junction of the pharyngeal clefts; equivalent ectoderm in the mammal may become associated with the cervical sinus and this can sometimes be implicated in the formation of part or all of the epithelium of a definitive cervical thymus.

In mammals the thymic anlage is associated with the region of the 3rd and 4th pharyngeal pouch, the major contribution coming from pouch III. Unlike other vertebrates it is the ventral part of the pouch, not its dorsal area, which gives rise to the developing thymus (see figure 4.1 and figure 7.3). The thymus of the adult mammal, including that of the monotremes, has a typical structure comprising a number of lobules, each with a cortical and medullary zone.

Role of the thymus. The function of thymus-derived T-cells is discussed in section 1.8.4. Much of this information comes from experiments on thymectomized mammals, especially those on mice. These experiments leave no doubt as to the essential role of the thymus in the maturation of full immune capabilities. Animals thymectomized at a sufficiently early stage of development frequently show severe immunological defects. Congenital absence of the thymus in man (Di George syndrome) and in mice of the "nude" strain similarly leads to crippling of the cellular immune system. On the other hand, early thymectomy in foetal sheep and in the pouch young of marsupials has a somewhat different outcome. Thus removal of the thymus from the sheep foetus at 60–70 days of gestation does not disturb the vigour of skin allograft reactivity in later life, nor does it affect the growth of the animal, or its ability to form circulating antibodies. These findings still hold when treatment with antilymphocytic serum is combined with foetal thymectomy, and they remain true for sheep thymectomized as early as day 48 of foetal life, when the thymus has only been lymphoid for some 5 days. These sheep do, however, show diminished delayed hypersensitivity reactions and a long-lasting deficiency in the number of circulating lymphocytes, although with an eventual slow recovery of normal lymphocytic levels.

A prolonged deficiency of lymphocytes also occurs when the thymus is removed from the very immature pouch young of marsupials; indeed this seems to be a consistent finding in early thymectomized animals in general. Quokkas thymectomized before 20 days of pouch life show decreased responses in delayed hypersensitivity reactions and to *in vitro* stimulation with phytohaemagglutinin (PHA). They grow well but have a shortened life span. These animals are eventually able to reject skin allografts and to synthesize antibody to various antigens (sheep erythrocytes, bacteriophage and *Salmonella adelaide* flagellae). Both the cellular and the humoral immune responses are slow to develop in the thymectomized quokka, but they finally appear and are effective by the time the juvenile is about 5 months old. From experimental evidence such as this, it has been suggested that an alternative pathway exists for the differentiation of at least some part of T-cell function and that, in the absence of the thymus, cells with the appropriate immune capabilities can be spawned in other tissues, albeit by a sluggish process requiring many weeks for completion.

Secondary lymphoid organs

In the monotremes (echidna) the spleen has a peculiar triradiate shape but otherwise resembles the spleen of the higher mammals. The secondary lymphoid organs which show most advancement, both in architecture and in number, within the class Mammalia are the lymph nodes. The lymph nodes of marsupials and eutherians have a complex architecture which is distinctive of the higher mammals; those of the monotremes are more simple in structure. In monotremes (in echidna and in the platypus *Ornithorhynchus*), each node appears to represent a single lymphatic nodule, whereas the lymph nodes of marsupials and eutherians contain a number of lymphatic nodules grouped within the node in the cortex. They also have a distinct medullary region which is absent in monotremes.

In the lymph nodes of higher mammals, afferent vessels bring lymph into the subcapsular sinus, whence it percolates through radial sinuses which converge eventually into large efferent vessels. In monotremes, on the other hand, several separate lymphatic nodules (of about 0·2–2·0 mm diameter) lie scattered within the lumen of a lymphatic plexus. Each is suspended by a vascular bundle from the wall of the vessel and is therefore bathed in lymph (figure 9.2). The nodules contain germinal centres (usually one per nodule). These resemble the germinal centres in the eutherian node, and they respond in the same way to antigenic stimulation. Thus, in the echidna, radio-labelled *Salmonella adelaide* flagellar antigen can be traced to the germinal centre where it becomes localized, often in the form of a cap similar to the specialized antigen-trapping region of the lymphatic nodules in eutherians. Radio-labelled *Salmonella adelaide* flagellar antigen can be located in only some of the lymphatic nodules of a cluster. Possibly in the higher mammals the multifollicular lymph node has an advantage over the anatomical arrangement in monotremes, particularly in terms of secondary exposure to antigen, in that each time the lymph-borne antigen percolates through the eutherian node, the majority (if not all) of the follicles are likely to encounter it.

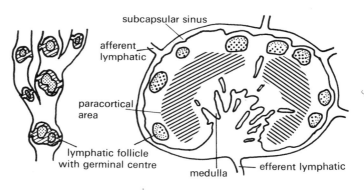

(a) *Monotreme*   (b) *Eutherian mammal*

**Figure 9.2.   Schematic diagram comparing the lymph nodes of mono-
tremes and of higher mammals**

(a) In monotremes, several separate lymphatic nodules (follicles) with
their germinal centres lie within the lumen of a lymphatic plexus;
each is suspended by a vascular bundle from the lymph vessel wall.

(b) In Eutherian mammals, in contrast, the lymph node is multifollicular: a number of lymphatic nodules lie within the cortex of
the single node and the afferent lymphatic vessels run into a
subcapsular sinus which surrounds the whole node.

Diagram (a) from Diener, E., Ealey, E. H. M. and Legge, J. S. (1967).
"Phylogenetic Studies on the Immune Response III. Autoradiographic
Studies on the Lymphoid System of the Australian Echidna *Tachy-
glossus aculeatus*", *Immunology*, **13**, 339–347 (with modifications).

Diagram (b) partly after Humphrey, J. H. and White, R. G. (1970),
Immunology for Students of Medicine, 3rd ed., F. A. Davis Company,
Philadelphia.

In non-mammalian vertebrates, even when lymph nodes occur, they are not numerous: the simple lymph nodes of the advanced anurans are relatively few in number; in birds, if macroscopically visible lymph nodes are present at all, they comprise only 2–6 pairs. In mammals, on the other hand, lymph nodes are abundant. Even in the opossum they are quite plentiful; over 20 nodes (mostly paired) are found in the North American species *Didelphis virginiana*, and 40 have been counted in the South American opossum *Didelphis azarae*. These opossum lymph nodes occur singly, one at each lymphatic drainage site of the region. Bats are similar to marsupials in this respect, but the majority of eutherian mammals display a multiplicity of lymph nodes, at least at some of the sites. This is particularly obvious in the larger eutherians—there are about 450 altogether in man. The effect of having multiple nodes in a single drainage area is that the lymph is filtered more efficiently; e.g. if there is a string of three nodes, the lymph is triple-filtered through macrophage-lined sinuses between its entry and its exit from the region, which may be advantageous, particularly where the fluid volume is large.

Thymectomy experiments in quokkas indicate that thymus-dependent areas occur in the secondary lymphoid organs of marsupials, located (as in eutherians) in the periarteriolar regions of the splenic white pulp and in the paracortical zone of the lymph nodes. Anatomical variations may occur in lymph nodes within the Eutheria. Some nodes filter blood as well as lymph (haemolymph nodes); these are especially abundant in ruminants. In the pig the node is inverted, the "medulla" being located at the periphery. Newborn pigs which are kept germ-free and deprived of colostrum, lack plasma cells and germinal centres in their secondary lymphoid organs. Such animals provide a useful model in which to study the effect of antigenic stimulation on lymphoid-tissue differentiation and antibody production, and have shown that large pyroninophilic cells appear in response to primary immunization, and that germinal centres are not a prerequisite of the response but are formed as a result of it; the germinal centres probably play a role in secondary immune responses.

9.2. Conclusions

The immune system of monotremes is in some respects intermediate between the reptilian condition and that of higher mammals, although it is distinctly mammalian in the structure of its IgG molecules and in most aspects of its lymphoid-tissue structure. In so far as they have been studied, marsupials seem to parallel the eutherians; e.g. in the possession of an

IgE-like immunoglobulin class. Their peculiar reproductive physiology (which may be their undoing in evolutionary terms) apparently leads to very slow maturation of immunocompetence during ontogenetic development. Some of the other deficiencies in immune capabilities described in marsupials relate to the opossum and may, in part, reflect the primitive and interesting status of this animal rather than genuine differences between marsupials and eutherians, especially since relatively little work has been done on the more primitive species of eutherian mammals.

Homoiothermy and viviparity are major advancements. Homoiothermy provides an evolutionary incentive for increased efficiency of the immune system in mammals as in birds. Viviparity involves complex maternal/ foetal relationships; the long period for which the young is protected may permit a build-up of cellular populations within the immune system before functional commitments need be made. This may aid in the acquisition of functional heterogeneity, a feature which typifies the mammalian immune system and which permits sharp discrimination, efficient specializations and refined feedback mechanisms. These complex reactions and interactions occur within the anatomical framework of the lymphoid tissues. Of these, the mammalian lymph nodes represent, in effect, an evolutionary innovation, for they have advanced far beyond the rudimentary organs of other vertebrates. Their cytoarchitecture provides a highly structured microenvironment which is specialized to fulfil the complex functions of an advanced secondary lymphoid organ. Regional responses within the system of lymph nodes, added to those of the other secondary lymphoid organs, provide for discrete and well-controlled local reactions, while at the same time being part of a highly integrated total immune system. Heterogeneity and functional specialization also occur at the molecular level in the increased immunoglobulin repertoire of mammalian humoral immune responses and at the cellular level, e.g. in the subdivision of T-cell functions—although on this latter point we have as yet insufficient information about heterogeneity in non-mammalian systems.

CHAPTER TEN

SUMMARY AND COMMENTS

10.1. Phylogenetic perspectives

The animal kingdom comprises creatures of such diverse structure and habit that to expect to draw a straight line from "primitive" to "advanced" is as unrealistic for immune capabilities as for any other body functions. One should look rather for adaptive radiation at various levels of sophistication and for defence systems which are suited to the overall physiology and ecology of the animals concerned. Furthermore, studies to date have relied largely on a "mammal-based" technology whose methods, choice of antigen, timing and other parameters may not be those best suited to animals of a different class. To this must be added problems of husbandry, for many of the interesting species are difficult to obtain, house and rear. Nevertheless, a sufficient body of information is now emerging for trends to be apparent, and the purpose of this chapter will be to summarize these and to comment upon some of the more interesting unresolved questions of comparative immuno-biology.

10.1.1. *The evolution of immune capabilities*

The internal defence mechanisms of higher animals involve the complex integration of components which perhaps at first served functions not exclusively related to defence, and which probably had separate phylogenetic origins. Thus phagocytosis is already present in the protozoa, and is used by animals of all groups for a variety of purposes which can include nutrition and waste disposal, as well as protective functions. Specific reactions which involve cell surface receptors, and which distinguish self from non-self, are less relevant to protozoa than to multicellular animals, since the protozoan cell surface usually relates to the external environment rather than to cells of its own kind; nevertheless, protozoa treat "self" fragments differently from those of other species. Specific aggregation of cells from the same species is already demonstrable in the most primitive metazoans (the sponges) where it is associated with the elaboration of substances which can block the adherence of cells of a different strain. No damage to the non-self cells ensues, however, and the reaction seems more akin to phenomena involved in the aggregation of tissue cells of higher vertebrates than to immune responses.

Incompatibility reactions (as opposed to aggregation phenomena) are first seen in coelenterates. These involve a primitive type of cell-mediated immunity which discriminates between self and non-self, and which can effect quasi-immune hyperplastic reactions leading to death of non-syngeneic cells. These reactions lack a memory component, but they may be analogous to the blastogenic response which occurs in the vertebrate mixed lymphocyte reaction. Secondary immune responses arise with the advent of true circulatory systems. This is probably no mere coincidence, since the circulation of body fluids not only disseminates potential pathogens, but also assists the movements of cells capable of recognizing them, thus making secondary encounter a more likely event. Cell-mediated immunity clearly precedes humoral antibody production in phylogeny. It is present in invertebrates of both the protostome and deuterostome lines, a fact which implies either a very early origin of cell-mediated immunity or convergent evolution in these two distinct superphyla. The question of homology or analogy will probably be resolved when more is known of the receptor molecules on the surface of cells which effect specific immunoregulation. The major question, as yet unresolved, is whether these invertebrate receptor molecules are related to vertebrate immunoglobulin (in which case, invertebrates have failed to take the next important step of secreting the product) or whether they are some different recognition molecule, with possible affinities to one or more of the complex array of circulating humoral factors found in diverse invertebrate animals.

On present evidence, immunoglobulin appears to be a vertebrate invention and, furthermore, one which brings with it an increased efficiency of response. The improvement may be partly at the recognition level (although fine discrimination also occurs in some invertebrates), but it could operate at the stage after recognition, the stage at which the immunocompetent cell is triggered to divide and amplify the response. Amplification, in terms of increased numbers of immunocompetent cells, occurs in invertebrates as well as in the vertebrates and, in both groups, the capacity to be triggered can function independently of the specific receptors, as well as through their agency; nevertheless, clonal expansion is impressive in vertebrates and undoubtedly makes an important contribution to the overall efficiency of their immune responses.

10.1.2. *Transplantation reactions*

The fact that transplantation reactions are generally slow in invertebrates and memory appears to be of limited duration may relate not only to primitiveness *per se*, i.e. to variations in the ability to recognize "foreignness" and to be triggered by it, but also in the amount of "foreignness" which is there to be recognized. Thus groups may differ in the strength and spectrum of the histocompatibility antigens which they possess. Also, in some experiments, the potential histocompatibility differences within the species may not be fully represented in the sample which is tested, especially when animals captured from the wild are taken from restricted geographical areas. Further limitations in poikilotherms may occur at the anatomical level (e.g. there may be poor connections with the graft area) and ambient temperature will also play its part. Moreover, there may be interaction with humoral factors. Thus in some vertebrate transplantation experiments (especially where histocompatibility differences are weak) the outcome can involve a delicate balance between cytotoxicity and enhancing antibodies.

In many animals (even perhaps in the simple aggregation of sponge cells) there is evidence that a single genetic region controls the major histocompatibility reactions. This region becomes increasingly polymorphic and, in higher vertebrates, is linked to other capabilities, such as immune responsiveness. The advantage of this latter form of genetic control remains, at present, speculative. Strong histocompatibility antigens and rapid rejection are features associated with the more advanced vertebrate groups.

10.1.3. *Humoral immunity*

Humoral antibody production based on the immunoglobulin molecule occurs only in vertebrates; and the essential features must have evolved early in their phylogeny, since almost all vertebrates can produce immunoglobulins with the basic 2H-2L heavy-chain and light-chain structure. The only deviation from this pattern is seen in the Agnatha, where lamprey immune molecules may consist of heavy (μ-type) chains held together by non-covalent bonds. IgM immunoglobulins are present in all gnathostomes, and their heavy chains show a high degree of similarity. There is also substantial conservation of light-chain structure. Furthermore, all vertebrates respond to a wide array of antigens, and this suggests an early origin of the variable region of the immunoglobulin molecule. The antiquity of IgM and the selective forces maintaining its occurrence throughout the vertebrates, probably relate to the role that this type of immunoglobulin plays in forming a cell surface receptor for antigen, the receptor being a single unit (7S) IgM. Polymeric humoral IgM with its multiple binding sites, may well have been the form best suited to the needs of early vertebrates (in which most immune responses take place on a local basis). In the more advanced animals, physiological changes (e.g. those involving high-pressure blood vascular systems) may have provided the evolutionary incentive for further adaptations, namely those leading to the production of low-molecular-weight antibodies and to new classes and subclasses of immunoglobulin with specialized biological functions.

Primitive features of the humoral antibody responses of lower vertebrates include less diversity of the immunoglobulin classes and, where low-molecular-weight antibodies are elicited, a slow and incomplete switch to their production. The ability of antibodies bound to antigen to fix complement is present in all jawed vertebrates, indeed the full complement system and the 2H-2L antibody molecule seem to have arisen at about the same time in evolution.

Vertebrate humoral immunity based on immunoglobulins by no means replaces more ancient defence mechanisms such as phagocytosis. On the contrary, it becomes increasingly linked to them, with inter-relationships at all stages from processing of the antigen to its final elimination. What is not clear is the antiquity of this link-up, by which recognition molecules come to impose a fineness of discrimination upon defence mechanisms with intrinsically low specificity. We can only note that analogous opsonizing agents also occur in some invertebrates.

10.1.4. *Lymphoid tissues*

Cells implicated in the internal defences of invertebrates include those resembling lymphocytes, granulocytes and macrophages. Lymphocytes are key cells in vertebrate immunology but, unfortunately, they are difficult cells to identify morphologically, since as "carriers of information" they comprise simply a nucleus and sufficient cytoplasm (usually just a small rim) to enable them to move; their small size assists penetration between cells. They are usually identified on nuclear features, unless distinctive immunological reactivity occurs (as in the case of tunicate lymphocytes) or immunoglobulin is detected. Invertebrate cells which resemble lymphocytes on morphological criteria alone, may prove instead to be wandering cells with the capability to develop along completely different lines.

In invertebrates, and in agnathans, there is as yet little evidence of any hierarchy of tissues which produce the immunologically competent cells (i.e. first-level, second-level and third-level organs as defined in section 1.7.1). Indeed, the clear demonstration of cell-mediated and humoral antibody responses in agnathans (which lack a distinct thymus and definitive lymphoid tissues) indicates that immunological capabilities do not depend on sophisticated lymphoid architecture. A functional distinction between cells concerned with cell-mediated immunity (T-cells) and those which produce humoral antibody (B-cells) may well exist in agnathans but, if so, we do not know whether at this stage in evolution they already form two distinct lines with separate developmental origins.

All the jawed vertebrates possess a primary lymphoid organ (the thymus) which retains a remarkably similar histology throughout the vertebrate classes (although its embryological origin may be from different pharyngeal pouches); they also have specialized secondary lymphoid organs, such as the spleen. Insertion of a primary lymphoid organ which is regulated by internal factors has an obvious evolutionary advantage in a system where, throughout life, the final stages of lymphocytic differentiation are governed by exogenous antigen. It is still questionable, however, whether the presence of the thymic epithelium, once evolved, is obligatory for the differentiation of T-cell function, or whether it merely provides a specialized microenvironment which quantitatively expands the number of T-cells produced by the animal and/or permits a further stage of maturation. The notion that vertebrates may be capable of some T-cell differentiation in the absence of the thymus comes from the results of certain thymectomy experiments (see section 9.1.4). Similar arguments have been applied to the avian bursa of Fabricius with regard to B-cell differentiation. The question may well be resolved when the role of possible humoral secretions by the epithelial components of the primary lymphoid organs is firmly established.

The *in vitro* responses of lymphocytes show a striking similarity in most of the vertebrate classes. Recent evidence points to a heterogeneity in these reactions among the lymphocytic populations of poikilotherms which, by analogy with mammalian T-cell and B-cell functions, would suggest an early evolution of this major dichotomy. There is a strong possibility that the heterogeneity will, as in mammals, prove to be linked to the organ of origin, i.e. that it will be thymus-dependent or thymus-independent, but this has yet to be established experimentally.

In poikilothermic vertebrates, much of the lymphoid tissue occurs in organs with sinusoidal blood flow, such as the kidney and liver, and the primitive lymph nodes of amphibians. These may provide sites where lymphoid cells can cluster and respond to the presence of antigen. Moreover, in tissues where the blood flow is slow, this is possibly all that is required. The development of elaborate lymphocyte migratory pathways is perhaps related to the more efficient circulation of body fluids, when architectural modifications within the lymphoid organs may have become necessary in order to ensure that cells can move in and out of the circulation at appropriate sites. Some of the apparent simplicity of the lymphoid organs of poikilothermic vertebrates may therefore be related to general features of the animals' anatomy and physiology rather than to deficiencies in immune potential.

At the cellular level also, antibody responses of the lower vertebrates, which are occurring on a dispersed and local basis, can be effected by antibody-forming cells which are relatively unspecialized morphologically. In higher vertebrates, on the other hand, the evolution of high-pressure blood systems, together with closed metanephric kidneys, may have eliminated a lot of areas which were previously suitable for local antibody production. This perhaps led to the evolution of the mammalian type of lymph node, and to the emergence of specialized trapping sites, complex germinal centre formation and a greater emphasis on the plasma cell which is geared to produce a large quantity of antibody. These plasma cells first appear in chondrichthian fishes, but considerable structural modifications are apparent in the more-advanced vertebrates.

10.1.5. *Diversity in the higher vertebrates*

Specialization at all levels—of immunoglobulins, of cell types, of T-cell and B-cell functions, and of microenvironments—is apparent in the mammalian immune system, and to a large extent also in that of birds. It is tempting to relate at least some aspects of this diversity to the amniote condition. Thus, when larvae are free-living, foreign antigens may be encountered when the lymphoid system is still very immature, and this may necessitate a rapid maturation of the pathways which lead to positive immune responses, perhaps at the expense of more advanced differentiation. In the amniote embryo, on the other hand, the need to produce immunocompetent cells is less urgent, which may allow a further build-up of cellular populations before functional commitments need be made. This, and homoiothermy, may have provided strong drives towards increased sophistication and diversity of the immune potential.

There remains the possibility that some of the differences between the repertoires of homoiothermic and poikilothermic vertebrates are apparent rather than real, since the amount of effort devoted to the study of mammalian systems is of a different order of magnitude from that expended on poikilotherms. Nevertheless, the diverse functional and morphological specializations, the high level of integration, and the carefully controlled feedback mechanisms which characterize mammalian organization in general, are also apparent in the immune system and typify the defence mechanisms of higher vertebrates.

FURTHER READING

A. THE IMMUNE SYSTEM (Chapter 1)

(a) Textbooks

Abramoff, P. and La Via, M. (1970), *Biology of the Immune Response*, McGraw-Hill Book Company, New York.

Bellanti, J. A. (1971), *Immunology*, W. B. Saunders Company, Philadelphia.

Boyd, W. C. (1966), *Fundamentals of Immunology*, Interscience, London.

Burnet, F. M. (1969), *Cellular Immunology*, Cambridge University Press.

Carr, I. (1972), *Biological Defence Mechanisms*, Blackwell Scientific Publications, Oxford.

Eisen, H. N. (1974), *Immunology: An Introduction to Molecular and Cellular Principles of the Immune Responses*. Reprinted from Davis, Dulbecco, Eisen, Ginsberg and Wood's *Microbiology* (2nd ed.), Harper and Row Publishers Inc., Hagerstown, Maryland.

Holborow, E. J. (1973), *An ABC of Modern Immunology* (2nd ed.), Little, Brown and Company, Boston.

Humphrey, J. H. and White, R. G. (1970), *Immunology for Students of Medicine* (3rd ed.), Blackwell Scientific Publications, Oxford.

Kabat, E. A. (1968), *Structural Concepts in Immunology and Immunochemistry*, Holt, Rinehart and Winston Inc., New York.

Park, B. H. and Good, R. A. (1974), *Principles of Modern Immunobiology: Basic and Clinical*, Lea and Febiger, Philadelphia.

Roitt, I. M. (1974), *Essential Immunology* (2nd ed.), Blackwell Scientific Publications, Oxford.

Steward, M. W. (1974), *Immunochemistry*, Chapman and Hall, London.

Weir, D. M. (1973), *Immunology for Undergraduates* (3rd ed.), Churchill Livingstone, Edinburgh and London.

(b) More specialized books, symposia, reviews and general articles

Amos, B. (Ed.), (1971), *Progress in Immunology*, *1*, Academic Press, New York and London.

Beer, A. E. and Billingham, R. E. (1974), "The embryo as a transplant". *Scientific American*, **230**, 36–46 (April).

Billingham, R. E., Brent, L. and Medawar, P. B. (1956), "Quantitative studies on tissue transplantation immunity. III. Actively acquired tolerance", *Philosophical Transactions of the Royal Society, Series B*, **239**, 357–414.

Brent, L. and Holborow, J. (1974), *Progress in Immunology*, *2*, North Holland Publishing Company, Amsterdam.

Burnet, F. M. (1959), *The Clonal Selection Theory of Acquired Immunity*, Cambridge and Vanderbilt University Press.

Cooper, M. D. and Lawton, A. R. III. (1974), "The development of the immune system", *Scientific American*, **231**, 58–70 (November).

Cottier, H., Odartchenko, N., Schindler, R. and Congdon, C. C. (Eds.), (1967), *Germinal Centres in Immune Responses*, Springer-Verlag, Berlin.

Diener, E. (1970). "The primary immune response and immunological tolerance", *Handbuch der Allgemeinen Pathologie*, **7**, part 3, 250–325, Springer-Verlag, Berlin.

Edelman, G. M. (Ed.), (1974), *Cellular Selection and Regulation in the Immune Response*, Raven Press, New York.

Elves, M. W. (1966), *The Lymphocytes*, Lloyd Luke, London.

Good, R. A. and Fisher, D. W. (Eds.), (1971), *Immunobiology*, Sinauer Associates Inc., Stamford, Connecticut.

Good, R. A. and Gabrielsen, A. E. (Eds.), (1964), *The Thymus in Immunobiology*, Hoeber-Harper, New York.

Greaves, M. F., Owen, J. and Raff, M. (1973), *T and B Lymphocytes: Their Origins, Properties and Roles in Immune Responses*, North Holland Publishing Company, Amsterdam.

Jerne, N. K. (1973), "The immune system", *Scientific American*, **229**, 52–63 (July).

Lindahl-Kiessling, K., Alm, G. and Hanna, M. G. Jnr. (1971), *Morphological and Functional Aspects of Immunity*, Plenum Press, New York and London.

Marchalonis, J. J. (Ed.), (1975), *The Lymphocyte: Structure and Function*, Marcel Dekker Inc., New York (in press).

Mayer, M. M. (1973), "The complement system", *Scientific American*, **229**, 54–66 (November).

Metcalf, D. and Moore, M. A. S. (1971), *Haemopoietic Cells*, North Holland Publishing Company, Amsterdam.

Miller, J. F. A. P. and Osoba, D. (1967), "Current concepts of the immunological function of the thymus", *Physiological Reviews*, **47**, 437–520.

Nelson, D. S. (1968), *Macrophages and Immunity*, North Holland Publishing Company, Amsterdam.

Nossal, G. J. V. and Ada, G. L. (1971), *Antigens, Lymphoid Cells and the Immune Response*, Academic Press, New York and London.

Porter, R. R. (1967), "The structure of antibodies", *Scientific American*, **217**, 81–90 (October).

Porter, R. and Knight, J. (Eds.), (1972), *Ontogeny of Acquired Immunity*, Ciba Foundation Symposium, Elsevier, Amsterdam.

Rogers Brambell, F. W. (1970), *The Transmission of Passive Immunity from Mother to Young*, North Holland Publishing Company, Amsterdam.

Rose, N. R., Milgrom, F. and van Oss, C. J. (Eds.), (1973), *Principles of Immunology*, Macmillan, New York.

Sercarz, E. E., Williamson, A. R. and Fox, C. F. (Eds.), (1974), *The Immune System. Genes, Receptors, Signals*, Academic Press, New York and London.

Smith, R. T. and Good, R. A. (Eds.), (1969), *Cellular Recognition*, Appleton-Century-Crofts, New York.

Solomon, J. B. (1971), *Foetal and Neonatal Immunology*, North Holland Publishing Company, Amsterdam.

Turk, J. L. (1967), *Delayed Hypersensitivity*, North Holland Publishing Company, Amsterdam.

Weiss, L. (1972), *The Cells and Tissues of the Immune System*, Prentice Hall Inc., Englewood Cliffs, New Jersey.

Yoffey, J. M. (Ed.), (1967), *The Lymphocyte in Immunology and Haemopoiesis*, Edward Arnold, London.

B. COMPARATIVE ASPECTS (Chapters 2–10)

(a) Phylogeny and ontogeny of immunity

American Society of Zoologists (1975), "Developmental Immunology", *American Zoologist*, **15**, 1–213.

Burnet, F. M. (1971), " 'Self-recognition' in colonial marine forms and flowering plants in relation to the evolution of immunity", *Nature*, London, **232**, 230–235.

Clem, L. W. and Leslie, G. A. (1969), "Phylogeny of immunoglobulin structure and function", pp. 62–88 in Adinolfi, M. (Ed.), *Immunology and Development*, Spastics International Medical Publications, London.

Cooper, E. L. (1975), *Comparative Immunology*, Prentice Hall Inc., Englewood Cliffs, New Jersey (in press).

Du Pasquier, L. (1974), "The genetic control of histocompatibility reactions: phylogenetic aspects", *Archives de Biologie*, **85**, 91–103.

Hildemann, W. H. (1972), "Phylogeny of transplantation reactivity", pp. 3–73 in Kahan, B. D. and Reisfeld, R. A. (Eds.), *Transplantation Antigens: Markers of Biological Individuality*, Academic Press, New York and London.

Hildemann, W. H. (1974), "Some new concepts in immunological phylogeny", *Nature*, London, **250**, 116–120.

Hildemann, W. H. and Cooper, E. L. (Eds.), (1970), *Symposium on the Phylogeny of Transplantation Reactions. Transplantation Proceedings*, **11**, 179–341.

Kampmeier, O. F. (1969), *Evolution and Comparative Morphology of the Lymphatic System*, C. C. Thomas Publishers, Springfield, Illinois.

Marchalonis, J. J. (1974), "Phylogenetic origins of antibodies and immune recognition", pp. 249–259 in Brent, L. and Holborow, J. (Eds.), *Progress in Immunology, 2*, volume 2, North Holland Publishing Company, Amsterdam.

Marchalonis, J. J. (Ed.), (1975), *Comparative Immunology*, Blackwell Scientific Publications, Oxford (in press).

Smith, R. T., Good, R. A. and Miescher, P. A. (Eds.), (1967), *Ontogeny of Immunity*, University of Florida Press, Gainesville.

Smith, R. T., Miescher, P. A. and Good, R. A. (Eds.), (1966), *Phylogeny of Immunity*, University of Florida Press, Gainesville.

Société Française d'Immunologie (1972), *L'Étude Phylogénique et Ontogénique de la Réponse Immunitaire et son Apport à la Théorie Immunologique*, Symposium: Paris.

(b) Invertebrate defence mechanisms

Acton, R. T. (1974), "Primitive recognition systems", pp. 287–291 in Brent, L. and Holborow, J. (Eds.), *Progress in Immunology. 2*, volume 2, North Holland Publishing Company, Amsterdam.

Cohen, E. (Ed.), (1974), "Biomedical perspectives of agglutinins of invertebrate and plant origins", *Annals of the New York Academy of Science*, **234**, 1–412.

Cooper, E. L. (Ed.), (1974), *Contemporary Topics in Immunobiology*: volume 4: *Invertebrate Immunology*, Plenum Press, New York and London.

Federation of American Societies for Experimental Biology: Pathology Symposium, (1967), "Defense reactions in invertebrates", *Federation Proceedings*, **26**, 1664–1715.

Hildemann, W. H. (1974), "Phylogeny of immune responsiveness in invertebrates", *Life Sciences*, **14**, 605–614.

Hildemann, W. H. and Reddy, A. L. (1973), "Phylogeny of immune responsiveness: marine invertebrates", *Federation Proceedings*, **32**, 2188–2194.

Jackson, G. J., Herman, R. and Singer, I. (Eds.), *Immunity to Parasitic Animals*: volume 1, Part 3: "Immunity of Invertebrate Hosts", pp. 111–228, Appleton-Century-Crofts, New York.

Laboratoire de Zoologie et Centre de Morphologie Expérimentale du C.N.R.S., Institut de Biologie Animale, Avenue des Facultés, 33-Talence (1971). "Colloque sur les reactions immunitaires chez les invertebrés", *Archives de Zoologie expérimentale et générale*, **112**, 55–116.

Salt, G. (1970), *The Cellular Defence Reactions of Insects*, Cambridge University Press.

Uhlenbruck, G. (1974), "Invertebrate immunology", pp. 292–296 in Brent, L. and Holborow, J. (Eds.), *Progress in Immunology. 2*, volume 2, North Holland Publishing Company, Amsterdam.

(c) **Comparative vertebrate immunobiology**

Aitken, I. D. (1974), "Avian immunology", pp. 302–307 in Brent, L. and Holborow, J. (Eds.), *Progress in Immunology*. 2, volume 2, North Holland Publishing Company, Amsterdam.

Ambrosius, H., Hemmerling, J., Richter, R. and Schimke, R. (1970), "Immunoglobulins and the dynamics of antibody formation in poikilothermic vertebrates (Pisces, Urodela, Reptilia)", pp. 727–744 in Sterzl, J. and Riha, I. (Eds.), *Developmental Aspects of Antibody Formation and Structure*, Volume 2, Publishing House of the Czechoslovak Academy of Sciences, Prague, Academic Press, New York.

American Society of Zoologists (1971), *Symposium on the Biology of Immunity in Amphibians, American Zoologist*, **11**, 167–237.

Anderson, D. P. (1974), *Fish Immunology*, TFH Publications Inc. Limited, Hong Kong.

Avtalion, R. A., Wojdani, A., Malik, Z., Shahrabani, R. and Duczyminer, M. (1973), "Influence of environmental temperature on the immune response in fish", *Current Topics in Microbiology and Immunology*, **61**, 1–35, Springer–Verlag, Berlin.

Cohen, N. (1975), "Phylogenetic emergence of lymphoid tissue and cells", in Marchalonis, J. J. (Ed.), *The Lymphocyte: Structure and Function*, Marcel Dekker Inc., New York (in press).

Cooper, E. L. (1973), "The thymus and lymphomyeloid system in poikilothermic vertebrates", pp. 13–38 in Davies, A. J. S. and Carter, R. L. (Eds.), *Contemporary Topics in Immunobiology*: volume 2, *Thymus Dependency*, Plenum Press, New York and London.

Cooper, E. L. and Du Pasquier, L. (1974), "Primitive vertebrate immunology", pp. 297–301 in Brent, L. and Holborow, J. (Eds.), *Progress in Immunology*. 2, volume 2, North Holland Publishing Company, Amsterdam.

Du Pasquier, L. (1973), "Ontogeny of the immune response in cold-blooded vertebrates", *Current Topics in Microbiology and Immunology*, **61**, 37–88, Springer-Verlag, Berlin.

Fichtelius, K. E., Finstad, J. and Good, R. A. (1968), "Bursa equivalents of bursaless vertebrates", *Laboratory Investigation*, **19**, 339–351.

Glick, B. (1970), "The bursa of Fabricius: a central issue", *Bioscience*, **20**, 602–604.

Good, R. A., Gabrielsen, A. E., Peterson, R. D. A., Finstad, J. and Cooper, M. D. (1966), "The development of the central and peripheral lymphoid tissue: ontogenetic and phylogenetic considerations", pp. 181–206 in Wolstenholme, G. E. W. and Porter, R. (Eds.), *Thymus: Clinical and Experimental Studies*, Ciba Foundation Symposium, Churchill, London.

Good, R. A. and Papermaster, B. W. (1964), "The ontogeny and phylogeny of adaptive immunity", *Advances in Immunology*, **4**, 1–115.

Goodman, J. M. and others (collected works), (1972), *Phylogenetic Development of Vertebrate Immunity II*, MSS Information Corporation, New York.

Grey, H. M. (1969), "Phylogeny of immunoglobulins", *Advances in Immunology*, **10**, 51–104.

Jackson, G. J., Herman, R. and Singer, I. (Eds.), (1969), *Immunity to Parasitic Animals*: volume 1. Part 4: "Immunity of cold-blooded vertebrates", pp. 231–275; volume 2. Part 5: "Immunity in avian hosts", pp. 295–420; volume 2. Part 6: "Immunity in mammalian hosts", pp. 421–1134, Appleton-Century-Crofts, New York.

Kubo, R. T., Zimmerman, B. and Grey, H. M. (1973), "Phylogeny of immunoglobulins", pp. 417–477 in Sela, M. (Ed.), *The Antigens*, volume 1, Academic Press, New York and London.

Marchalonis, J. J. and Cone, R. E. (1973), "The phyl'enetic emergence of vertebrate immunity", *Australian Journal of Experimental B. 'ogy and Medical Science*, **51**, 461–488.

Mizell, M. (Ed.), (1969), *Biology of Amphibian Tumours*, Sp. ger-Verlag, Berlin.

Wang, A. C. and Fudenberg, H. H. (1974), "IgA and evolutic of immunoglobulins", *Journal of Immunogenetics*, **1**, 3–31.

INDEX

INDEX